SOCIAL SKILLS TRAINING FOR CHILDREN WITH ASPERGER SYNDROME AND HIGH-FUNCTIONING AUTISM

Social Skills Training
for Children with
Asperger Syndrome
and High-Functioning Autism

SUSAN WILLIAMS WHITE

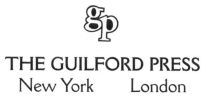

THE GUILFORD PRESS
New York   London

© 2011 The Guilford Press
A Division of Guilford Publications, Inc.
72 Spring Street, New York, NY 10012
www.guilford.com

Printed in the United States of America

This book is printed on acid-free paper.

Last digit is print number: 9   8   7   6   5   4   3   2   1

The author has checked with sources believed to be reliable in her efforts to provide information that is complete and generally in accord with the standards of practice that are accepted at the time of publication. However, in view of the possibility of human error or changes in behavioral, mental health, or medical sciences, neither the author, nor the editor and publisher, nor any other party who has been involved in the preparation or publication of this work warrants that the information contained herein is in every respect accurate or complete, and they are not responsible for any errors or omissions or the results obtained from the use of such information. Readers are encouraged to confirm the information contained in this book with other sources.

Library of Congress Cataloging-in-Publication Data

White, Susan Williams.
    Social skills training for children with Asperger syndrome and high-functioning autism / by Susan Williams White.
        p. cm.
    Includes bibliographical references and index.
    ISBN 978-1-60918-209-0 (cloth: alk. paper)
    1. Social skills—Study and teaching.   2. Asperger's syndrome.   3. Autism in children.   I. Title.
    HQ783.W515 2011
    362.196′858832—dc22
                                                                                    2011009165

About the Author

Susan Williams White, PhD, is Assistant Professor of Psychology at the Virginia Polytechnic Institute and State University (Virginia Tech), where she codirects the Virginia Tech Autism Clinic. She is also a clinical psychologist specializing in the treatment of people affected by neurodevelopmental disorders such as the autism spectrum disorders (ASD). Dr. White is currently conducting a treatment study, funded by the National Institute of Mental Health, on high-functioning adolescents with ASD who also struggle with anxiety. She has written extensively on assessment and treatment considerations for people with ASD and has a special interest in interventions for social deficits and co-occurring psychiatric problems, such as anxiety in individuals with ASD.

Acknowledgments

This book draws not only from my own clinical work and research experience but also from the wealth of knowledge generated by many dedicated scientists and clinicians who have committed their professional lives to helping people affected by autism and related conditions. I cannot possibly be so thorough as to thank all of them individually, as I would like to do. However, I would like to acknowledge the invaluable consultation I have received from some of the most influential and generous individuals with whom I have had the good fortune to work. Dr. Lawrence Scahill, my postdoctoral advisor at the Yale University School of Medicine Child Study Center, has shaped my thinking about developmental disorders and taught by example how to integrate good science with ethical clinical care. I have also had the good fortune to work closely with Drs. Ami Klin, Connie Kasari, Cynthia Johnson, and Donald Oswald—professionals who have helped countless individuals and families with autism spectrum disorders (ASD) through their direct clinical work and research. I would like to thank Kathleen Koenig, MSN, also of the Yale Child Study Center, who has conducted social skills groups for children with ASD for several years and has been instrumental in developing novel strategies and techniques for teaching specific skills.

This book would never have been possible had it not been for the families and patients with whom I have interacted over the years. I am grateful for their willingness to work with me and their commitment to their treatment goals. Thinking of their struggles and of how hard they persevere makes me keep striving when I feel frustrated by setbacks or what seem to be unsolvable problems. I thank my husband, Bradley, and my two sons, Alden and Calvin, both of whom were born during the writing of the book! Having you in my life is both a grounding influence and a constant source of inspiration.

I would like to extend a sincere thank-you to Dr. Anne Marie Albano, who motivated me to write this book. Dr. Albano's insightful feedback challenged me to dig deeper into some of the unique clinical complexities involved in working with families affected by autism. And, finally, thanks to Senior Editor Kitty Moore of The Guilford Press for her editorial support.

Contents

CHAPTER 1

Introduction

I wrote this book for clinicians, teachers, and others who want to help children and teenagers affected by autism spectrum disorders (ASD) to improve their social skills. This clinical guide offers practical approaches and suggestions for teaching social skills to children and teenagers with autism and related conditions. Once regarded as rare, more recently these disorders have received a great deal of scientific and media attention as a result of rising prevalence estimates. In 2009 the United States Centers for Disease Control and Prevention (CDC) reported that spectrum disorders are as common as 1 in every 110 people (CDC, 2009). Given the current prevalence estimates and the empirically supported importance of early identification (Dawson, 2009), we undoubtedly face a growing, and aging, ASD population. *The fastest-growing area of need, in terms of ASD and mental health, is likely to be with older children, adolescents, and adults.*

Many clinicians, including those who do not specialize in treating people with ASD, are being asked to work with patients who desperately need some type of help with impaired social functioning. The number of families seeking treatment far exceeds the available clinical resources in most communities. School systems are also being called on to serve a growing student population identified as having either autism or a related condition and therefore needing special services. Most schools are relatively unprepared to deal with this growing demand, and school officials are unsure of how best to meet the needs of students with ASD and their families. This problem is by no means limited to specialists or special education teachers. On the contrary, many students with higher-functioning forms of ASD are served almost exclusively by regular education teachers and are taught the general educational curriculum. Thus, the onus is placed on regular education teachers, many of whom have had little or no training on working with students with ASD.

Most therapists and mental health clinicians have some familiarity with social skills training as a treatment approach for a variety of childhood disorders and problems. It is a commonly used approach in the treatment of many childhood disorders. Nevertheless, social skills training is generally not effective as the *sole* form of intervention for most psychiatric or behavioral disorders (e.g., Spence, 2003). It is but one component of a comprehensive intervention program that may include therapy, school consultation, and sometimes medication. This approach is also standard when working with individuals who have autism spectrum conditions. In individuals with ASD, the social disability may be viewed as fundamental—or the common impairment threading across all spectrum disorders—but it nevertheless is related to many other factors and aspects in the person's life. Treatment should therefore be integrated, building appropriate prosocial skills and addressing as many related factors (e.g., communication impairments, hyperactivity, over-selectivity) as possible. Thus, let me offer a word of caution for readers of this guide: *although social skills training is generally best viewed as an important component in any comprehensive treatment program for a child with ASD, it should typically not be the only type of treatment provided.*

This guide represents an attempt to address a growing need in the mental health care and educational communities, to assay current thinking in this area, and to disseminate potentially useful approaches for social skills training for children and teens with ASD. As such, the material in this book draws from multiple theoretical approaches, clinical interventions, and treatment models. It does not represent any single social skills training curriculum. In integrating material from multiple sources, I have sought to provide clinicians and teachers with a resource that provides both conceptual and hands-on material, enabling the practitioner to decide which approaches best fit the needs of the particular client with whom he or she is working. Both mental health clinicians—that is, psychologists, therapists, social workers, and school psychologists—and educators—including both regular education and special education teachers as well as school counselors—should be adequately prepared to treat these children and their families now and into the foreseeable future.

What Is ASD?

The disorders collectively known as ASD are neurodevelopmental conditions typically diagnosed early in childhood. The exact etiology of these disorders is unknown. Although genetic factors are generally accepted as being at least predisposing factors, there are likely multiple genes involved and myriad pathways that can lead to a final diagnosis of an ASD. It is also probable that spectrum disorders arise from a variety of sources, meaning that no single cause underlies all cases of ASD or autism. Furthermore, there may be genetic predispositions that can be triggered by environmental or developmental insults or events that may make possible the subsequent development of the ASD. This diversity in ontology probably helps to explain the variability seen in people with ASD. Individuals on the autism spectrum can and do look very different from one another in every way imaginable—language ability, intelligence, sense of humor, interests, desire for human closeness, and prognosis, to list just a few.

Regardless of cause, all spectrum disorders are characterized by deficits in social interaction. The other two core domains of interest are communication deficits and the presence of repetitive behavior and restricted interests (*Diagnostic and Statistical Manual of Mental Disorders* 4th Ed., text revision [DSM-IV-TR]; American Psychiatric Association, 2000). A person's behavioral profile in the communication and restricted behavior/interests domains influences specific ASD diagnosis. In early childhood, for example, an adolescent with high-functioning autism likely was delayed in developing spoken language, whereas one with Asperger syndrome may have been precocious in terms of language development or at least not delayed. There is also some evidence for wide differences in learning profiles with respect to visual–spatial abilities and verbally mediated skills. However, as stated previously, *all of these disorders are characterized by deficits in social interaction*. Problems with communication, both verbal and nonverbal, and stereotyped behavior and/or restricted interests are diagnostically informative but are not the defining features of the spectrum disorders.

A Word on ASD Subtypes

"Autism spectrum disorders" is a term that encompasses three related neurodevelopmental conditions: autistic disorder, Asperger syndrome (AS; also known as Asperger's disorder), and pervasive developmental disorder not otherwise specified (PDD-NOS). The distinction between high-functioning autism (HFA) and AS typically does not determine the type of social skills intervention chosen. However, there are some general characteristics unique to each group[1] that may affect how one intervenes to effectuate change in social skills. Diagnostically, autistic disorder precludes a diagnosis of AS—they cannot coexist. AS is distinguished by the absence of intellectual disability or the delayed development of spoken language. In adolescents who are higher-functioning (i.e., within the range of normal cognitive functioning, or not mentally retarded), differential diagnosis of HFA and AS may be difficult. There is some empirical evidence that youths with AS tend to be "active but odd" in their social interaction attempts as compared to those with HFA, who tend to be more aloof and passive (Ghaziuddin, 2008). In other words, children with AS may be more likely to initiate inappropriately (e.g., ask personal questions), intrude into the personal space of another person, and be more socially impulsive and naïve. On the other hand, those with HFA might respond appropriately to questions asked about themselves but not feel the need to reciprocate, or ask questions of conversational partners.

In practice, the latter group may be more difficult to carry on a conversation with, while with the former it may be difficult to get a word in edgewise! When one or the other of these characteristic sets is present, it will determine the type of intervention implemented. A sense of social deficit pervades all ASD subtypes, regardless of how intellectually gifted the person may be.

As this book goes to press, we face proposed changes in the next edition of the DSM (DSM-5) that will substantially affect how we conceptualize the spectrum conditions (see *www.dsm5.org/Pages/Default.aspx*). These changes may make much of the difficulty surrounding specific subtype diagnosis a thing of the past. "Autism spectrum disorder" will be the diagnostic label for individuals now labeled as having autistic disorder, AS, childhood disintegrative disorder, or PDD-NOS. The separate diagnostic labels (e.g., AS) will no longer be applied, as they are absorbed into the single spectrum condition. These changes, largely based on a lack of data consistently supporting a clear distinction between mild autistic disorder and AS, are not universally supported. For instance, in a 2009 *New York Times* article, Dr. Simon Baron-

---

[1]Making broad generalizations about characteristics associated with an ASD subtype is difficult because of the tremendous individual variability within the diagnostic subtypes. There will always be exceptions, when such generalizations are made. Nevertheless, knowing the "typical" characteristics associated with a subtype can be helpful in treatment planning, as long as knowledge of the individual client supersedes any such generalization.

Cohen (2009) asserted that scientists are just now beginning to identify biological and genetic markers associated with AS, a relative newcomer to the diagnostic scene, first included in the DSM-IV in 1994.

Despite the proposed changes to our diagnostic system, the specific profile of social deficits presented by the client can be useful in determining *how* to deliver the intervention. For instance, intervention with a child who is socially aloof and essentially uninterested in his peers and friendships will look quite different from intervention with a child who is highly socially motivated but naïve and awkward around his peers. As the mental health profession moves toward a more holistic view of ASD, distinguishing specific diagnoses within the spectrum will become a thing of the past. Because the HFA–AS distinction does not drive the choice of social skill intervention(s) and in light of the move toward a more unified view of autism spectrum disorders, *the term "ASD" is used throughout this book to refer to people with HFA, AS, and/or PDD-NOS.*

Why Focus on Social Skills Development?

Socialization deficits are a major source of impairment regardless of cognitive or language ability for individuals with ASD (Carter, Davis, Klin, & Volkmar, 2005), and they do not remit with development. Indeed, impairment and distress may increase as the child approaches adolescence, when the social milieu becomes more complex and demanding, and as the individual becomes more aware of his or her social disability or "differentness" (Schopler & Mesibov, 1983; Tantam, 2003). Owing to this increasing self-awareness and the growing social complexity associated with middle childhood, social skills deficits may presage mood and anxiety problems later in development (Myles, 2003; Tantam, 2003), especially among higher-functioning individuals with ASD. The importance of social interaction and having a group of friends in which one feels accepted and supported is often overlooked, or taken for granted, by people without a severe social disability.

Social acceptance affects the overall quality of life and, for teens especially, has an impact on academic functioning and developing identity and self-worth. Indeed, social difficulties in ASD have been found to be linked to multiple other problems. Although it is often assumed that individuals with ASD prefer to be alone and have little social contact, many people with ASD are intensely aware of their isolation and unhappy about their lack of connectedness with others (Attwood, 2000). Moreover, clinical reports indicate that deficits in social interaction may lead to more serious problems, specifically anxiety and mood disorders, as children with ASD mature. Both teens and adults with ASD are at increased risk for depression and anxiety (Ghaziuddin, Weidmar-Mikhail, & Ghaziuddin, 1998), which can negatively impact academic and social performance (Myles, Barnhill, Hagiwara, Griswold, & Simpson, 2001). A self-awareness of social deficits, emotional isolation, and secondary problems with depression can be detected in these two statements made by adolescents with ASD:

- "Asperger's is the reason why my friends are paid to take me places by my parents."
- "Because I have Asperger's I always have to worry about my social skills, and I can mess up really badly at any time."

Finally, it is generally accepted by behavior analysts and psychologists that all behaviors are purposeful. If the drive for social interaction is present but the child lacks the knowledge and capacity to use appropriate social skills to satisfy this drive, he or she will probably begin to apply more socially *inappropriate* behaviors to get this need or drive met. For example, if a high school girl cannot figure out how to be accepted by peers in class in the same ways that the other girls are accepted (e.g., by talking about topics of mutual interest, such as current television shows), she may find that acting up or telling inappropriate jokes gets her some amount of peer attention. And although such behaviors may successfully garner attention, they also often lead to such unintended consequences as school detention as well as eventual rejection or further isolation from peers. The point of this example is that if the drive is present but the requisite skill (knowledge of and fluency in skill use, or the like) is not, other less desirable behaviors will likely be called on to satisfy the drive.

To summarize:

- Socialization problems are the key defining feature of all ASD subtypes.
- For cognitively higher-functioning individuals with ASD, socialization problems often stem *not* from lack of motivation but rather from lack of ability.
- Social skills deficits are associated with other problems, including anxiety, depression, and further isolation, that impede the child's success and quality of life.

For all these reasons, it is logical to make social skills training a focus of treatment for children and teens with ASD.

Why Target "High-Functioning" Youths?

As previously discussed, there is considerable heterogeneity among people with ASD. The level of cognitive functioning, or intelligence, is one area that can vary greatly among youths on the autism spectrum, affecting how treatment is delivered and what is targeted within any social skills intervention program. Higher-functioning adolescents with autism spectrum conditions have been found to initiate social interaction with peers more frequently than do their lower-functioning peers with ASD. Their rate of social initiations, however, is still about half that of their typically developing (non-ASD) peers (Bauminger, Shulman, & Agam, 2003). Teens with ASD also tend to receive fewer social initiations, or bids inviting action(s), from their peers. *Both minimal social initiations on the part of the person with ASD and lack of opportunity to respond appropriately to the initiations of others likely affect social functioning to its detriment.* Given that a general lack of *knowledge and skill* of how to initiate social actions (or reciprocate or interact, etc.) rather than a lack of *desire* underlies teens' perceived social isolation and loneliness, it is imperative that they are taught *how* to initiate interactions more frequently and more effectively.

This guide focuses on social skills training approaches for school-age children and adolescents with ASD who are considered "high-functioning," typically defined as individuals without severe cognitive impairment. In most research literature, the term "high-functioning" refers to people with ASD whose assessed Full Scale IQs fall at or above the borderline range (i.e., IQ $\geq$ 70) and, usually, who are able to communicate verbally. The reason for focusing on this specific group of individuals, as defined functionally, is that doing so affects the specific types of interventions undertaken. Children who do have co-occurring intellectual disability can learn more appropriate social skills, but the approaches used to teach individuals with significant cognitive and verbal limitations are *qualitatively different* from those that can and should be used with individuals without such limitations. Individuals with co-occurring intellectual disability may require more intensive adult prompting and visually based rather than verbally based teaching strategies. In teaching social skills to an adolescent with comorbid intellectual disability, for instance, one might include modeling appropriate social skills based primarily on simple visual aids (e.g., cartoon pictures) and also provide tangible reinforcers to help motivate skill practice. As you will see, for example, many of the strategies in this guide are verbally mediated or require a fair amount of instructor modeling and self-reinforcement.

With respect to the decision to focus on school-age children and older subjects (i.e., ages 7–17), the approaches one implements with a school-age child are qualitatively different from those undertaken with a very young child. The social play of very young children differs from that of school-age children in that there is more reliance on props and less social reciprocity; their social networks and friendships lack the complexity and depth seen in the peer groups of older children. Although some adaptation of teaching methods and content is necessary for teenagers, in general the approach to training or instructing a 10-year-old with ASD is fairly similar to that with a 15-year-old.

Despite being able to demonstrate average—or sometimes significantly above-average cognitive functioning—youths with ASD nonetheless generally manifest severe social limitations and impairments. Their unique cognitive profiles, combined with communication difficulties (e.g., monotone speech), contribute to difficulty in interacting in social situations as well as understanding and recognizing their own internal states. The social interaction difficulties encountered are profound and do not tend to improve developmentally without intervention. Difficulties with processing information about others, such as interpreting others' intentions and inferences, lie at the heart of the social difficulties characteristic of ASD. Adolescents with ASD typically have great difficulty in understanding the social expectations of their peers, knowing how to act in unstructured situations (e.g., a school field trip), and adapting their behaviors to fit the demands of the situation. Compounding these inherent social skills deficits, problems with emotion regulation and overarousal all too often amplify the subjects' impairments.

Although people with ASD, especially those with AS, do not necessarily have a problem with speaking, difficulties with the most basic practices of social communication are characteristic concerns. Recognizing how nonverbal cues such as a person's tone of voice or intonation can alter the intent and interpretation of a spoken communication is often problematic. So is understanding nonliteral language, such as irony or sarcasm. The social communication of individuals with ASD is further hampered by such problems as not knowing how much information to provide, not readily providing contextual cues to help the listener make sense of the topic of conversation, and often making tangential or off-topic comments (Twachtman-Cullun, 1998).

In summary, youths with spectrum disorders uncomplicated by intellectual disability should not be viewed as less severely affected by social deficits than those with classic autism or severe cognitive limitations. In fact, their heightened self-awareness during later childhood and adolescence and their desire to interact with peers likely *compound* their social deficits over time. For this reason, and also owing to the differences in teaching approaches discussed earlier, this guide focuses on higher-functioning youths.

Overview of Social Skills Training

"Social skills training" is a term used to describe a broad class of interventions designed to remedy interpersonal skill deficits. All of these interventions share the goal of improving children's social competence, usually as a means of promoting adjustment and decreasing impairment. There is no single unifying theoretical approach that underlies all social skills training approaches. However, the basic assumption is that social competence is related to attaining and maintaining satisfying social relationships, which in turn are related to an improved quality of life (Segrin & Givertz, 2003).

Unlike many of the skills children are taught, like how to brush one's teeth or ride a bicycle, social skills are almost entirely context-dependent. As opposed to more *concrete* skills, social skills rely on unwritten "codes of conduct"—that is, they vary depending on the situation, the people one is with, what just happened, and what is about to happen. Even more perplexing for individuals with ASD who can typically learn and follow set rules very well is the fact that social skills change over time. For instance, a 4-year-old may learn that he or she should approach other children as potential playmates and politely ask, "Do you want to be my friend?" This is a fine skill for a 4-year-old, but when the boy or girl is 13, that same social skill is no longer appropriate. This difference helps to convey why social skills training interventions are so difficult, namely, it is hard to nail down a moving target!

Gresham, a pioneer in the field of social skills training, has differentiated three types of social skills deficits: skills acquisition deficits, performance deficits, and fluency deficits (Gresham, Sugai, & Horner, 2001). A *skills-acquisition* deficit conveys that the child lacks the know-how for performing a given skill. A *performance* deficit is present when the child has the knowledge but fails to demonstrate the skill when it is needed. Finally, a *fluency* deficit is present when the child knows the skill and is motivated to do it well but "renders an awkward or unpolished performance of the social skill" (Gresham et al., 2001, p. 334). *The type of deficit indicated should determine what type of intervention is done*, whether it be teaching the skill, prompting its use, or practicing and rehearsing the appropriate skill in a natural setting. Consider the examples provided in Table 1.1, which describes some of these deficit types as they might be expressed in a child with ASD.

Most social skills programs follow a similar teaching sequence (e.g., Evans, Axelrod, & Sapia, 2000). After first assessing the child's functioning to determine which specific social skills to target, the skill(s) are taught—often in a small-group format with same-age peers. Following the didactic instruction, the child gets the opportunity to prac-

TABLE 1.1. Types of Skill Deficits

Type of deficit	Examples	Intervention possibilities
Acquisition	1. Child does not know what cues indicate it is okay to talk to someone (e.g., person smiles at you). 2. Child lacks understanding of how nonverbal behaviors (e.g., a smile, a wave of the hand) communicate emotions.	Teaching discrete skills in a one-on-one or group format
Performance	1. Child does not initiate conversations at school despite demonstrating the skill during sessions with the therapist. 2. Child verbalizes an understanding of the importance of nonverbal communication, yet fails to use facial expressions or gestures while speaking.	Integrating teaching within the child's classroom; involving other peers, siblings, etc.
Fluency	1. Child interrupts others to start a conversation about topics that are not of interest to peers. 2. Child stares at peers when speaking and waves hand emphatically when approaching someone in greeting—almost to the point of touching the peer.	Providing feedback on skill performance; modeling appropriate execution of the skill

tice the skill in a semistructured setting (e.g., in the training group) before attempting to transfer the skill to the child's natural environment (e.g., school) to promote generalization. In addition to teaching skills that the child is either lacking (acquisition) or has difficulty performing well (performance or fluency deficit), most approaches also attempt to reduce competing or other problematic behaviors (Gresham, Thomas, & Grimes, 2002).

What We Know from Non-ASD Populations

There is empirical evidence supporting a relationship between success-ful social relationships, or *social competence*, and psychological health (Parker & Asher, 1987; Greene et al., 1999). Moreover, social skill defi-cits are associated with the development and diagnosis of many childhood psychiatric disorders (Hansen, Nangle, & Meyer, 1998). Social skills interventions have been implemented for the treatment of most childhood disorders and problem behaviors, including attention-deficit/ hyperactivity disorder (ADHD) (de Boo & Prins, 2007), depression (Segrin, 2000), aggression (Nangle, Erdley, Carpenter, & Newman, 2002), and shyness (Greco & Morris, 2001). Behavioral approaches—by far the preferred methodology of most social skills training approaches— include such strategies as modeling, role play, rehearsal, providing feedback to the child, real-world practice, and reinforcement.

Models of ASD Social Dysfunction

Social skills training is often a core component of treatment programs for youths with ASD for whom social skill deficits are the fundamental problem. I make no attempt to cover all of the theoretical models and scientific conceptualizations proposed to explain the various social dysfunctions seen in ASD. However, an overview of some of the primary theories can help shape our understanding of the social skills deficits frequently seen in this population. For more information on these theories, the interested reader is directed to Carter et al. (2005) or to the research underlying these orientations that is provided in this volume's references.

The most widely espoused theory for explaining ASD social dysfunction is probably theory of mind (ToM), or mindblindness, proposed by Baron-Cohen (1995). According to ToM, social deficits result primarily from an inability to consider and conceptualize one's own mental phenomena as well as those of others. This basic shortcoming makes it especially difficult to predict or understand the intentions, feelings, and beliefs of others. Indeed, lack of understanding that a person has feelings, thoughts, and beliefs that do not always correspond to reality and an inability to attribute such thoughts to self or others make it quite difficult to make sense of or predict other people's behavior. Such deficits can make social reasoning impossible and social discourse overwhelming.

Consider the case of "Ben," a 15-year-old who is unable to appreciate that his classmates do not share his intense fondness for riddles and rhymes. In fact, not only do they not share his interest, but they also find it irritating that he insists on rhyming when he speaks up in class, and they tease him about it. Unfortunately, in Ben's case, he was able to recognize the teasing as such and was deeply hurt by it. His propensity to answer in rhymes—for instance, when responding to a question from the teacher—was so driven a compulsion that he felt powerless to refrain. Another example demonstrating impaired ToM is the middle school student "Ari," who has a crush on a girl in class, one that is not reciprocated. Ari tries talking to the girl, and eventually he even shares his feelings with her. The girl, wanting to spare his feelings, does not directly tell him that she likes a different boy. Instead, she politely tells him she appreciates his feelings and, when he asks her out time and again, finds convenient excuses to decline (e.g., "My family will be out of town then"). He persists in asking the girl out, totally oblivious that she is interested in someone else. In essence, Ari lacks any awareness of a tacit social rule that most young people "get" intuitively, namely, that multiple rebuffs of a social invitation usually indicate disinterest and that therefore he should desist. In both of these examples, the boys with ASD seem unaware of practical commonsensical knowledge that is collectively "shared" by their peers. To put it another way, they simply don't "get it," and this lack of insight sets them up for rejection and social humiliation.

A second theoretical model links social dysfluency to deficits in executive functioning (EF), a group of abilities that allows one to plan ahead, shift priorities, and act purposefully despite distractions or competing demands (Ozonoff, 1997). There are many specific abilities that fall within the EF domain; those that appear to be most impaired in children with ASD are related to flexibility and planning (Ozonoff & Jensen, 1999). Logically, deficits in EF could lead to some of the commonly seen problems in ASD, including poor application of formal knowledge to real-world problems, a tendency to perseverate (i.e., repeat actions or words) and difficulty in staying on task when working or interacting with others. Deficient EF characteristic of ASD might be best exemplified in commonly seen problems with adjusting to altered routines and unexpected changes. Consider a teenage girl who comes to English class prepared for the test she has studied for, only to be greeted by a substitute teacher announcing that the test will not take place today because the regular teacher is ill and she wants to use today as a review day. Most students can readily accept this change in plans and perhaps even be relieved by the realization that they have an extra day to study. This student, however, becomes very upset and dysregulated. She might react in a hostile way, perhaps yelling at the substitute teacher, or become very quiet and even more rigid (e.g., retreating to a corner to read her favorite book while rocking from side to side in her chair).

Weak central coherence (Frith, 2003; Happe, 1996), a third theoretical explanation, may also help elucidate the social deficits evident in ASD. This theory highlights problems with understanding the "meaning," or gestalt (whole picture) of things seen in many people with ASD.

An inability to attend to *context*, to integrate pieces into a central totality, underlies social deficits in individuals on the autism spectrum. In other words, successful social functioning necessitates that one integrate multiple pieces of context-dependent information, such as recognizing the relationships among various individuals, following the thrust of the conversation as it shifts from person to person, and such other factors as the time and environment—all at a very fast pace in order to respond appropriately. Children with ASD generally lack these abilities. There are many ways in which problems with synthesizing multiple pieces of information to inform the whole can detrimentally affect social functioning. Consider the teenager who attends only to the verbal message "Nice shirt!" without noting the facial expression (a smirk) or tone of voice (condescending) of the person making the comment—or even the fact that other students are laughing. The message a teenager with autism might take away from the exchange might be "this is a sincere compliment" when, in fact, quite the opposite message was intended.

Klin and colleagues (Klin, James, Schultz, & Volkmer, 2003) described the enactive mind (EM) model as postulating that people with ASD tend to possess a general orientation to *things* rather than *people*. Based in cognitive neuroscience, the EM model explains why some people with ASD may be quite intellectually gifted or knowledgeable in certain areas of expertise (e.g., telephone circuitry) and yet be severely impaired socially. In studies using eye-tracking technology, which permits the researcher to determine exactly what a person is attending to and noticing in the environment, it has been found that people with ASD tend to neglect nonverbal social cues such as eye contact and pointing (Klin, Jones, Schultz, Volkmar, & Cohen, 2002). A failure to notice such social cues as they occur naturally would inevitably contribute to frequent misperceptions or oversights relating to important social interactions and, of course prevent appropriate social responses. One person's subtle wink, for instance, can be quite salient—it might signify an inside joke or indicate that he or she was just kidding (i.e., "Disregard what I just said"). But a person with ASD, who might not attend to eye gaze patterns, would not perceive this information or assign any salience to it and would therefore have only the verbal communication on which to base his or her understanding of the situation.

At this time, no single theory is universally accepted as an explanation of the developmental course of social deficits observed across the full range of spectrum disorders. Each theoretical model has its own strengths and limitations, and it may be wise to draw on aspects of several of the models, especially as we learn more about the neurological underpinnings of ASD (South, Ozonoff, & McMahon, 2007). In conceptualizing why a student struggles to appreciate the fact that his peers have little interest in talking about his favorite topic—dot matrix printers, for example—principles from ToM may be useful (e.g., an inability to distinguish his own interests and thoughts from those of other people) and can guide intervention. With this student, the explicit teaching of such skills as inferring someone's thoughts based on his or her facial expressions or actions might be useful. In another example— say, in explaining to parents how their daughter can apparently effort- lessly commit to memory the titles and publishing information of her favorite book series and yet be unable to identify any of her classmates by name—the EM model might be more applicable. However, in many cases, the incredible variability observable among individuals who are on the spectrum in terms of level of social motivation and social skill may make adoption of any single theory to explain the social deficits of ASD difficult if not imprudent.

Specific Social Deficits of ASD

The types of skill deficits seen in children and adolescents with ASD are diverse. Fluency deficits are seen in many higher-functioning students with ASD who have received explicit training in social skills and want to do well but who struggle with performing the skills in a fluid and natu- ral way. However, acquisition and performance deficits are also seen. In addition to deficits in specific discrete social skills such as appropri- ately modulated eye contact, youths with ASD often have difficulty with more "fluid" skills such as noticing and sharing affective experience and perspective taking (Gutstein & Whitney, 2002). Deficits in these higher- level skills inhibit a person's ability to maintain age-appropriate friend- ships in adolescence, when peer relationships are expected to be based on reciprocity and a shared understanding of unspoken things held in common.

The variability seen in social functioning across people who have spectrum disorders cannot be overstated. This variability is one of the main reasons why applying "predetermined" programs to enhance social functioning can be challenging. However, some deficits are frequently seen and should generally be considered when assessing a child's social abilities. Following are some of the more common skill deficits in chil- dren and adolescents with ASD:

- *A failure to establish a shared reference point when conversing with others.* A person with ASD may *launch* into a topic of dis- cussion without providing enough—or even any—background information for his or her conversational partner.
- *Lack of consideration, understanding, or appreciation of social*

norms or "rules." This deficit can be seen in the awkward or abrasive way a teen with ASD might approach a stranger or respond in class when asked a question. The youth might come off as rude or irritable when, in fact, he or she just doesn't observe such typical social "niceties" as responding with a smile or refraining from making potentially offensive comments (e.g., "Wow—your hair looks awful today!").

- *Overreliance on "scripts" for conversation, or stereotypical expressions used without reference to the context.* A person with ASD may learn a rule for social exchange (e.g., greet others with a smile and handshake) and then apply that rule across all situations independent of the context (e.g., applying the rule at all social events, including funerals and school dances).
- *Difficulty in understanding the nature of friendship.* Many youths with ASD struggle with appreciating the concept that friends can be shared, that friendships are not monogamous relationships. This deficit may be related to previous negative experiences with peers, prior difficulties in making new friends, or anxiety about how to interact in social groups. It can lead to jealousy and/or aggression. Similarly, a child may consider a peer to be a friend when the relationship is not truly reciprocal. A teen with ASD might call a peer a "friend" simply because that person acts civilly toward him or her regardless of whether the peer actually initiates conversations or invites the teen with ASD to do anything outside of school.
- *Lack of respect for personal physical space.* Along with the motor clumsiness and coordination difficulties often present in ASD, it is common to see teens with ASD impose on adults' and peers' personal space. A female counselor treating a child on the spectrum might be surprised, for example, when the client suddenly hugs her—and perhaps too tightly—at the end of a session owing to a lack of appreciation of personal space conventions and potential sensory difficulties.
- *Misperceptions of others' intentions and social behavior.* Teens with ASD may believe they are being bullied or picked on when in fact they are not. Conversely, they may not recognize when they are being targeted in a joke.
- *Misinterpretation of the nonverbal aspects of communication,* such as one's tone of voice and facial expression. A person with ASD might fail to notice another person's shift in tone of voice, or they might perceive it but not recognize how it alters the communication (for example, by not realizing that the person is only joking).

While this list is by no means exhaustive, and it is unlikely that any single child possesses all of these deficits, it provides examples of some of the commonly seen social challenges presented to therapists and teachers who work with children and teens on the autism spectrum. A model of ASD social dysfunction is depicted in Figure 1.1. This figure may be used as a handout with families as a tool for explaining some of the social difficulties children with ASD typically encounter and how they arise.

Among people with spectrum disorders, those with better-developed verbal and cognitive abilities have been found to initiate more social interactions with peers (Sigman & Ruskin, 1999). However, their interactions are often awkward or sometimes even offensive. Teens with ASD, especially higher-functioning individuals, are likely to struggle to be accepted and to experience attendant distress related to their lack of requisite skills. They are usually not well integrated into the social networks of their peers (Chamberlain, 2002) and may in fact experience considerable loneliness (Bauminger & Kasari, 2000). Moreover, social communicative competence is associated with better long-term outcomes for people with high functioning forms of ASD (Marans, Rubin, & Laurent, 2000). Given that the motivation to interact with peers is typically present but the skills are deficient, explicit training in appropriate social skills is a reasonable treatment approach.

There is currently a great deal of interest and research in determining how effective social skills development interventions are for youths with ASD. In a meta-analysis of 55 single-subject studies of school-based social skills training interventions for students with ASD, Bellini and colleagues (Bellini, Peters, Benner, & Hopf, 2007) concluded that social skills training approaches were only minimally effective. In a comprehensive qualitative review of group-delivered social skills programs for children and teens with ASD, White and colleagues (White, Koenig, & Scahill, 2007) found that multiple methodological shortcomings (e.g., small sample sizes, inadequate tools for assessing change) in prior studies have impeded our ability to accurately assess effectiveness. There is agreement among scientists and clinicians alike that, although social skills instruction for ASD is a logical treatment choice, much more research is needed in addition to evidence-based treatment manuals focused on promoting the generalization and maintenance of the skills gained (White et al., 2007; Rao, Beidel, & Murray, 2008).

Although research examining the effectiveness of social skills interventions for children and adolescents with ASD is still in its infancy, social skills training as a general class of interventions is an established method of treatment for other disorders that has generated growing

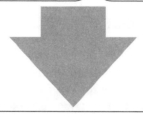

Theoretical Explanations of ASD Social Dysfunction

Theory of Mind Deficits: difficulty in understanding, appreciating, or inferring the mental and emotional states of self and others

Executive Function Deficits: poor planning and organizational skills, difficulty with flexibility

Enactive Mind: fixation on things rather than people, attention focused on nonsocial aspects of the environment

Weak Central Coherence: inability to conceptualize or integrate pieces into a whole or to make sense of context

SOCIAL SKILLS DEFICITS OFTEN SEEN IN CHILDREN WITH ASD:

- Difficulty in identifying and correctly interpreting one's own feelings and thoughts
- Inability to understand others' feelings, beliefs, intentions
- Lack of understanding as to why peers respond to them as they do (i.e., social cause–effect relationships)
- Inability to predict how others will behave or respond
- Tendency to perseverate on matters ("mental stickiness")
- Struggling to remain on topic in a conversation
- Inability to quickly assimilate social stimuli
- Tendency to overlook nonverbal aspects of social communication (e.g., eye contact, facial expressions)
- Tendency to ignore subtle social cues
- Frequent misinterpretation of others' behaviors
- Lack of appreciation for or understanding of nonliteral communication such as irony or sarcasm
- Tendency to perseverate on topic(s) of personal interest, regardless of others' lack of interest
- Frequent failure to provide sufficient background or context to conversational partners
- Rigidity and insistence that others follow "rules"
- Inability to apply social rules flexibly, once learned
- Social naiveté
- Tendency to be unintentionally blunt and at times socially offensive

FIGURE 1.1. Model of ASD social dysfunction.

empirical support (Mueser & Bellack, 2007). Such training has been integrated successfully into treatments for social phobia (e.g., Herbert et al., 2005; Bogels & Voncken, 2008) and schizophrenia in adults (Tenhula & Bellack, 2008; Granhom, Ben-Zeev, & Link, 2009), among other disorders and life problems. In summary, much is yet to be learned about how to most effectively improve social functioning in cognitively higher-functioning people who have ASD. Considerable progress, however, is being made in identifying promising strategies for improving the social functioning of youths with ASD. This volume provides readers with the relevant information on these supported and emerging strategies.

Organization of This Book

Sources of Material

Given that children with ASD fail to acquire age-appropriate social skills and usually lack opportunities for positive peer interactions, it is logical to assume that explicit instruction in social skills should be effective in helping them to be better prepared to succeed socially. Writing a clinically oriented book for practitioners and educators on social skills training approaches for ASD, however, is challenging in that there are no empirically supported treatment programs currently available. The logical questions to ask, therefore, are: "So, how do practitioners know what to do with patients on the spectrum who need such treatment?" and "What, then, goes into a guide on social skills training for ASD?" The content, suggestions, and related materials in this book derive largely from the current empirical research in the field as well as from clinical experience with this population and a basic theoretical understanding of these disorders. A great deal of research has been conducted in this area that has helped to shape our current understanding of what works best for whom. The general caveat addressed to readers of this guide, however, is that much of this research is preliminary and the conclusions tentative.

Our understanding of the effective treatment options for youths with ASD is still relatively early in its development. Not having a firmly "empirically supported treatment" for this clinical population, however, should not prevent us from treating kids who clearly need help based on what empirical evidence is available. As solid research continues to be carried out in this field, we must provide services to the best of our abilities by utilizing the knowledge and research that are thus far available. We must also inform our patients and their families about the limitations of our current clinical knowledge, including what is and is not known about the effectiveness of the treatments we provide. With this type of full disclosure, the clients we serve can make informed decisions about how they want to invest their time and resources in treatment.

Interventions based on the principles of applied behavior analysis have been successful for many children with ASD in improving communication deficits and reducing interfering and repetitive behaviors. Therapeutic interventions targeting social deficits, however, have not yet met with the same level of success. Indeed, social skills deficits remain the paramount treatment challenge for practitioners who work with individuals on the spectrum. In conclusion, the material in this book is derived from multiple sources including empirical data from peer-reviewed research studies and clinical trials, the available treatment manuals, professional experience with this population, the experience of colleagues who work in this area, anecdotal evidence, and my own theoretical knowledge of ASD. Where appropriate, the source of the information cited is provided. The interested reader is encouraged to gather additional information whenever possible on the specific approaches discussed.

Overview of the Chapters

Social skills training as an intervention approach has a long history in the field of mental health treatment. Accordingly, most practitioners who work clinically with children have a basic familiarity with many of the techniques traditionally used to teach social skills. Such knowledge can be very helpful in working with children on the autism spectrum. Many of the specific strategies covered in this book are adapted from research and clinical work on social skills training for non-ASD populations. Also, a solid knowledge base of typical social development during childhood and how nonautistic children interact with peers provides a good benchmark against which to compare the behaviors of our clients and students with ASD. The strategies in this volume have been modified for children and teens with ASD to help address learning difficulties or special challenges often seen in ASD. These modifications are highlighted within each chapter, and examples of successful implementation of the specific strategies are offered.

The chapters in this volume cover a broad range of practical information and suggestions for social skills training for youths with ASD. The chapters are divided topically as follows:

- Chapter 1. The theory and background of social skills training; key aspects of the primary social difficulties associated with ASD.
- Chapter 2. Clinical evaluation of social skills deficits in ASD; psychiatric concerns that can affect socialization.
- Chapter 3. An overview of the major types of interventions as well as significant adaptations made in delivering social skills instruction to youths with ASD.
- Chapter 4. Social skills training approaches used in group therapy.
- Chapter 5. School-based social skills training approaches; interventions that can be implemented in the inclusive classroom.
- Chapter 6. Strategies intended primarily for use in a clinical setting.
- Chapter 7. Promoting social skills training in children at home; overcoming common obstacles that affect social functioning.
- Chapter 8. Planning beyond childhood; addressing social competence in later adolescence and adulthood.

At the end of the book, suggested resources for further information, organized topically, are included in the section titled "Further Reading." The Appendix contains several blank forms that can be photocopied and adapted as needed by practitioners. Throughout the book, numerous case examples are offered to demonstrate client problems and intervention strategies. When the examples are based on real cases, all identifying information has been changed. The forms and worksheets may be photocopied for readers' use in practice or modified as needed to address the social skills difficulties that your specific client or student faces.

In conclusion, social skills training should typically not be the *sole* intervention used to treat an individual with ASD, as other interventions (such as medication, individual therapy, or parent training) are also needed to address each client's unique concerns. However, social skills training is a practical solution for addressing the primary social deficits characteristic of spectrum disorders. Social skills training has been applied to many other childhood problems and psychiatric disorders with mixed success. However, there are two important "givens" relating to children's social skills and their overall mental health:

1. *Deficient social interaction skills are associated with poorer functioning and mental health outcomes.*
2. *Social competence is associated with better overall adjustment and successful outcomes.*

These two principles hold true for individuals with ASD, as they do for neurotypicals.

Case Example

By the age of 12, "Samantha" had been hospitalized owing to aggression three times. Each hospitalization was preceded by an aggressive incident toward her family or peers. She was diagnosed previously with bipolar disorder and ADHD and had previously been prescribed several different medications.

In the sixth grade in a public middle school, Samantha was educationally classified as emotionally disturbed and had an individualized education plan. She was primarily taught in regular education classes, with some help for math. She typically did well in school academically but had more difficulty socially. Samantha had received social skills instruction throughout elementary school as part of her school's curriculum. Her parents reported no social concerns during her early elementary years, noting that Samantha interacted with peers appropriately, her parents set up many playdates for her, and she had several friends at school.

During her fifth-grade year, however, she began having problems with some other girls in her class. Samantha complained that they picked on her and called her names. She reacted by telling the teacher, or sometimes she would rush out of the class, crying and asking to go home. The problems escalated into the sixth grade, and Samantha began reacting more aggressively—destroying property and threatening peers.

Upon meeting with and observing her, the school psychologist concluded that Samantha was applying tactics or skills used by *younger* children in interacting with same-age peers. For example, after lunch outside she approached peers on three occasions, asking "Do you want to play with me?" The girls she approached on the first two occasions were not engaged in playing, but rather were just sitting near each other and were talking. On the third occasion, the two girls Samantha approached were reading books silently next to each other. On each occasion, Samantha reacted negatively—either yelling at the girls or running away. On the third occasion, she became destructive and began kicking in lockers.

After referral and a comprehensive evaluation, Samantha was diagnosed with Asperger syndrome. The school psychologist began seeing Samantha after school regularly and had daily "check-ins" with her between classes. Samantha struggled with emotion regulation and had many social skill deficits. She was often unable to express her emotions appropriately to peers and also had difficulty in interpreting the affective cues of others. She did not readily recognize when her own emotions were beginning to escalate, and she lacked practical strategies for regulating her emotions. She therefore typically overreacted and felt badly about it afterward, which left her feeling even worse about herself and lonely—thus exacerbating her social difficulties. The chosen treatment for Samantha addressed her emotion regulation as well as the teaching (skills acquisition) and practice (skills performance) of social interaction skills appropriate for adolescents.

CHAPTER 2

Clinical Evaluation and Assessment of Social Skills

This chapter focuses on assessment considerations and treatment planning. As discussed in Chapter 1, the socialization problems characteristic of ASD are pervasive and severely impairing. However, social skills deficits are typically not the *only* problem for children with ASD who present for clinical care. With a fair degree of regularity, clinicians and educators see children who also struggle with secondary psychiatric concerns. Such problems, when present, affect socialization and can impact the success of any social skills development intervention that is provided. Evaluating for other possible problems and diagnoses should therefore be part of the clinical intake and evaluation procedure. At the time of the initial evaluation, it is also advisable to consider how the changes in social skills will be assessed during treatment (i.e., monitoring treatment progress). This chapter covers both of these issues: the assessment of comorbid problems and the assessment of social skills deficits and the impact of treatment.

Secondary Clinical Concerns

A diagnosis of autism or AS does not preclude a diagnosis of most other psychiatric disorders in the same individual. It certainly does not prevent a child from struggling with other mental health issues, diagnostic criteria aside. However, many mental health concerns have a unique presentation in individuals with ASD. Some problems that are quite prevalent among people with ASD and can severely impair the person's functioning and development. Teachers and school personnel are often the first to recognize such problems (e.g., anxiety) in the school setting, and clinicians must address these types of problems in addition to social skills development. These problems can be severe enough to be the focus of intervention; even if they are not the main reason for clinical referral, they compound the social disability. If not addressed therapeutically, secondary problems to ASD often interfere with efforts to improve social skills. Consider, for example, a boy with generalized anxiety disorder (GAD) and ASD. In treatment, the boy struggles to learn the social approach strategies the therapist is teaching in response to his distraction and worry (e.g., about his health, his grades, his circumstances at home). In other words, his uncontrollable worries limit his ability to attend to new learning materials and "be present" during therapy. For these reasons, one must to consider secondary clinical issues when targeting social skills development. Summarized below are the most commonly related psychiatric diagnoses and difficulties.

Anxiety

People with ASD are highly susceptible to experiencing anxiety severe enough to adversely affect their normal functioning. Some anxiety is normal in everyone—even healthy and adaptive, under certain circumstances. Without "normal" anxiety, we might not be sufficiently vigilant while walking to our car at night in an empty parking lot, or we might approach strangers in a carelessly casual way. Anxiety that is chronic, uncontrollable, or disproportionate to the actual threat that is present (e.g., extreme fear of nonpoisonous spiders), however, becomes problematic. In a recent comprehensive review of studies on anxiety in youths with ASD, it was found that between 11 and 84% of children with ASD experienced impairing anxiety (White, Oswald, Ollendick, & Scahill, 2009); most estimates, however, fall between 40–45%. As is true with typically developing children, anxiety symptoms evolve over the course of development such that younger children on the spectrum are more likely to experience specific phobias, and older children and adolescents more often report symptoms of such disorders as obsessive–compulsive disorder (OCD) and social phobia.

A bidirectional relationship likely exists between anxiety and social deficits in ASD, and anxiety significantly amplifies the social impairments characteristic of ASD. For example, when anxious, a child with autism might abruptly withdraw from social situations, preferring to be alone. He might spend more time engaged in behaviors involving his own restricted personal interests and even become emotionally labile or irritable (e.g., Tantam, 2003). Social situations are especially anxiety-provoking for many young people with ASD because they lack appropriate social skills and are often acutely aware of their deficits (Kuusikko et al., 2008).

This sense of anxiety based on awareness can also contribute to what a colleague of mine refers to as the "freeze" response, in which the adolescent feels paralyzed to act in a social situation because she is so afraid of doing something wrong. *The teen's awareness of her own social difficulties, combined with a negative social learning history, makes her so anxious that she does not attempt to engage socially even when she possesses the ability to do so appropriately.* In such situations, having a few *brief and well-rehearsed scripts* or nonverbal social greetings (e.g., a smile and head nod) to call upon can be useful in "unlocking" the person so she can respond. Stress reduction techniques, such as deep breathing or calming imagery, can also be helpful. In other words, such a freeze response may be related to insight or awareness of one's own deficient social skills, and it is reality-based. Most young people with ASD have unfortunately experienced negative social exchanges with peers in the past such as victimization or bullying. If a young man has struggled with making friends in the past, knows he has a tendency to make odd or rude comments quite accidentally, and has experienced negative reactions (e.g., teasing), he may be unable to appreciate that he has subsequently developed more appropriate skills that he can actually use.

Unfortunately, problems with anxiety can often be difficult to identify or distinguish from the ASD diagnosis itself, because the symptoms and behaviors that may signal a problem with anxiety are not necessarily the typical types of behaviors indicative of anxiety disorders (e.g., exacerbation of repetitive behavior), and there is typically a lack of emotional insight on the part of the child (e.g., she may not identify feeling anxious or worried). Moreover, the linkages between anxiety and other ASD-related problems such as sensory sensitivities or repetitive behaviors can be difficult to pin down. A common concern is determining whether the behavior should be conceptualized as a repetitive feature of the ASD or rather as a compulsion linked to OCD complex.

When a comorbid anxiety disorder is present, I typically try to decrease the anxiety level before directly initiating the social skills development for two reasons. First, experiencing some degree of success during the early stages of treatment tends to bolster the child's confidence in herself and in the therapy and therapist, thereby increasing her "buy-in" to the treatment process. Once a child experiences success in overcoming a fear of elevators, for instance, it can make the very difficult job of learning and practicing improved social skills (e.g., appropriate responding to peers' teasing) a bit more tolerable, leading to more successful outcomes. Think of the task in this way: the social difficulties have been present throughout the child's life and are pervasive, whereas the anxiety problem, on the other hand, is usually more acutely felt and more immediately distressing. As such, the child may well have more motivation to do something about the latter problem. Noticeable improvement is also typically easier to achieve on anxiety problems in ASD than on the broad goal of improving social functioning. Second, the nature of the anxiety problem often mitigates against successful execution of even well-learned social skills, an observable phenomenon perhaps most true of comorbid social phobia. The young client strongly desires to improve his skills and works hard in therapy to acquire appropriate skills, and yet he fails to practice them outside of the session with peers because of his fear of negative evaluations from them.

It is not always the case that anxiety is targeted prior to social development, however. Sometimes, targeting improved social skills must go hand in hand with addressing the anxiety therapeutically, and in some cases it may take precedence. For example, if a child is working on exposures to address social anxiety, some basic social initiation skills might need to be inculcated therapeutically to make the exposures more successful. If the child is doing something socially inappropriate that would likely lead to peer rejection, for instance, addressing that behavior through detailed instruction should be tackled before encouraging additional social exposures.

Mood Disorders

Mood disorders may be especially common during adolescence in higher-functioning youth with ASD, probably owing in part to increasing self-awareness (Ghaziuddin et al., 1998; Myles, 2003; Tantam, 2003). In a recent study of adults with ASD, certain factors appeared to contribute to increased vulnerability to depression, including less severe social impairment, higher cognitive ability, and other psychiatric symptoms (Sterling, Dawson, Estes, & Greenson, 2008). A longitudinal study of new-onset psychiatric disorders in people with ASD, however, failed to find an association between childhood predictors of developmental outcome (i.e., intelligence, language) and the occurrence of secondary psychiatric disorders (Hutton, Goode, Murphy, Le Couteur, & Rutter, 2008). Nonetheless, treatment providers should be alert to the possibility that, as children with ASD experience social and cognitive improvement as a result of intervention, depressive symptoms may emerge (Sterling et al., 2008).

Bipolar disorder, characterized by periods of depression and mania, is sometimes diagnosed in children with ASD. There is, in fact, some evidence that bipolar disorder may be more prevalent than major depressive disorder among individuals with ASD (Munesue et al., 2008). Youths with ASD often present clinically as though the primary diagnosis is bipolar disorder (i.e., hyperarousal, emotional reactivity and dysregulation, and intense anger or aggression). Because they can quickly become upset and sometimes aggressive, often without an obvious external trigger, teenagers with ASD may be mislabeled as having bipolar disorder. On the other hand, it is entirely possible that both diagnoses are accurate. At this point, unfortunately, there is almost no empirical literature on the presentation and evidence-based differential diagnosis of bipolar disorder in ASD on which to base clinical decisions. Differentiation of the two conditions can be difficult. Limited insight, poverty of speech, alexythimia (the inability to access words to describe one's own emotions), and unusual emotional expression may all contribute to delayed identification of mood disorders secondary to ASD. Any suspicion of a mood disorder in ASD or the presence of long-standing social deficits in a child with depression should be further investigated and informed by a thorough family history and parental reports of changes in the child's emotions (Hutton et al., 2008; Matson & Nebel-Schwalm, 2007).

If symptoms of a mood disorder are present, the clinician needs to track the symptoms during the intervention. Depressive symptoms can undermine the success of social skills training—the client may feel hopeless about improvement, consistently fail to complete assigned between-session tasks, and/or engage in self-destructive behaviors. Moreover, given recent research indicating that the level of depression is related to the severity of ASD impairment, treating symptoms of depression directly may reduce ASD symptomatic impairment (Kelly, Garnett, Attwood, & Peterson, 2008). Similar to the priorities in treating a child with a co-occurring anxiety disorder, it may often be helpful to target reduction of depressive symptoms as an initial treatment goal. Behavioral activation and brief cognitive-behavioral therapy (CBT), for example, might be effective in reducing depressive symptoms and make the child more amenable to focusing on skills development. Medications can also be quite helpful in some cases. Regardless of the approach(es) taken, given the severity of some of the behaviors associated with mood disorders (e.g., self-harm, suicidal ideation), it is essential that such symptoms be closely monitored over the entire course of the intervention, even when the mood disorder is no longer the primary focus of clinical attention.

Attentional Problems

Children with HFA and AS tend to exhibit more symptoms of ADHD as compared to peers without ASD (Thede & Coolidge, 2007), and ADHD is probably the most common co-occurring condition in youths with ASD, especially prepubertal children (Ghaziuddin, et al., 1998). Sturm, Fernell, and Gillberg (2004) found that among children with ASD without comorbid intellectual disability, 95% had attentional problems and about 75% met the criteria for mild to severe ADHD. This finding occurred despite the fact that a diagnosis of autistic disorder disallows a dual diagnosis of ADHD (American Psychiatric Association, 2000). The DSM prohibits dual diagnosis of ASD and ADHD, because the symptoms of overactivity and inattention are so commonly seen in ASD. It has long been accepted that people with ASD usually have deficits in executive functioning skills in the areas of mental flexibility, impulse control, and inhibition (Pennington & Ozonoff, 1996). Children with AS, owing to their impulsivity and social disinhibition, are often initially diagnosed with ADHD in early childhood *prior to* identification of the ASD.

Some children with ASD and problems with inattention or hyperactivity can be helped with medication, such as methylphenidate, although the magnitude of their response is less than what is typically seen in children with ADHD and adverse effects (e.g., irritability) are more common (Research Units on Pediatric Psychopharmacology Autism Network [RUPP], 2005). Behaviorally based interventions and parenting/environmental interventions can also be helpful. Depending on the severity of the problem, symptoms of ADHD can make social skills interventions challenging and can decrease treatment success. A child with ASD and severe ADHD symptoms typically has a harder time attending during treatment sessions, grasping the material, and remembering how to use her skills in natural environments. For these reasons, accurate assessment of symptoms of ADHD at the outset of treatment is important. If symptoms are impairing, appropriate treatment and/or referral for medication may bolster the effectiveness of the social skills intervention.

In addition to co-occurring psychiatric disorders, other behavioral concerns can affect social skills use and social success at school. These problems do not necessarily represent diagnosable mental health disorders, but they do interfere with successful socialization with peers. Intellectual disability (i.e., mental retardation) is not included in this list, given that the focus of this book is on higher-functioning children with ASD. However, intellectual disability co-occurs in children with ASD, excluding those with AS, quite frequently. The CDC (2007) reported that between 33 and 58% of youths with ASD have cognitive impairment. The presence of intellectual disability will affect how intervention targeting social skills growth is delivered. Whenever a client presents with any of the following concerns, I try to integrate that particular concern into the treatment plan.

Socioemotional Immaturity

The social and emotional naiveté of school-age children and adolescents with ASD is striking. Even for clinicians and teachers who regularly work with youths on the autism spectrum, the lack of appreciation for age-appropriate social norms can be alarming. A teenager I once treated was in his high school's gifted and talented academic program. Both his extensive knowledge of mathematics and computational skills were impressive. However, he would frequently talk about his extensive Pokemon card collection with complete disregard for the fact that none of his peers had been interested in the cards for some time. Youths with ASD may say things that are out of keeping with their level of intellectual functioning and can often react quite immaturely. This pattern may be reflected in numerous aspects of the teen's life, such as poor self-care and hygiene skills, a lack of interest in such popular pursuits as dating or obtaining a driver's license, a relative absence of sexual curiosity, and only a rudimentary understanding of the nature of friendship.

Immaturity is typically especially evident in these adolescents' interest in and knowledge of sex and romantic relationships. Addressing the needs of adolescents with ASD as they relate to sexuality, dating, and interpersonal intimacy in general really does deserve its own chapter if not its own book! The problems presented clinically are highly diverse, to say the least. Many young people with ASD seem to have no appreciation for how sensitive such issues as sexual intimacy can be, while others seem over sexualized—bringing up personal topics when it's not appropriate to do so and using explicit language without necessarily any intent to offend; still others seem years behind their same-age peers in terms of sexual interest or knowledge. Unfortunately the research in this area is exceptionally sparse (Gabriels & van Bourgondien, 2007). In my own experience, I find it most helpful to ask about any problems with respect to interpersonal intimacy as early as possible in the therapeutic relationship. It is better to know whether such concerns/behaviors need to be addressed than to be surprised by some new development or unexpected remark once treatment is already well under way. If sexual immaturity issues are a treatment concern, the counselor needs to incorporate them into the treatment plan that addresses social skills development. While the sexual domain may arguably be the most sensitive of all to address, overlooking it does a disservice to the client and his or her family.

Especially during adolescence, sexuality and intimacy are important and developmentally appropriate concerns. Helping the young person to observe and take note of peers' behavior (e.g., how other boys typically talk about girls) can be educational in providing a basis for social comparison. Sometimes educational books or videos can provide the structured teaching needed. Of course, an appreciation for the values of the client's family, including their religious beliefs and family rules (e.g., about dating, and about a willingness to discuss sensitive issues), is important in this process. In treatment, the client needs to feel safe to ask questions of the counselor and discuss his or her concerns about sexuality. The same is true also for the parents, who often feel conflicted about what to do. On the one hand, they want their child to experience interpersonal happiness, enjoy satisfying relationships and ultimately love, and progress developmentally. Yet, on the other hand, parents of children with ASD normally harbor considerable fear about how their youngster will fare in this delicate area—and not without good reason. There is a real risk of both inappropriate actions on the part of the youth (e.g., acting upon a misinterpretation of another person's cues), which can lead to harm to others as well as possible legal problems, and victimization and sexual exploitation of the young person with ASD, given his or her severe social naïveté.

Anger and Aggression

Children who have autism and related conditions frequently exhibit such behavior problems as low frustration tolerance, temper tantrums, self-injury, and aggression toward others. Such behaviors can stem from multiple sources including environmental stimuli (e.g., sound sensitivity), demands placed upon the child, or internal stimuli (e.g., an untreated toothache). A recent study found that up to 27% of youths with ASD may meet the criteria for secondary diagnoses of oppositional defiant disorder (ODD), which is characterized by defiance toward authority and argumentativeness (Gadow, Devincent, & Drabick, 2008). Aggression may be more problematic for lower-functioning youths with ASD who lack the ability to express frustration or anger in more adaptive ways. Some pharmacological (i.e., risperidone; RUPP, 2002) and behavioral (e.g., RUPP, 2007) interventions have been helpful in reducing these problems. A structured behaviorally based parent training program designed to reduce noncompliant behavior was recently found to be acceptable to families, and preliminary results indicate its probable efficacy (RUPP, 2007). When such behavioral concerns are present, they usually need to be addressed *prior to* social skills improvement efforts, as such behaviors will clearly interfere with the use of appropriate skills and social integration.

Restricted Interests and Unusual Behavior Patterns

The third domain of behavior in the diagnostic criteria for autism is repetitive behavior or restricted interests. Children with ASD diagnoses vary a great deal in the degree to which this domain is prominent. When severe, repetitive behaviors can impede appropriate social skills use. A third grader who must repeatedly take his shoes off and put them on again in class, for example, cannot fully participate in class activities or interact with peers easily. Circumscribed but intense interests can have similar adverse effects on socialization. For instance, the middle school student with AS who is intensely interested in amphibians might initiate interactions with peers at school—but on closer examination it turns out that he always initiates them about his favorite topic (i.e., amphibians) *regardless of the interests of his conversational partners.* On the other hand, a child might not be highly verbal about special interests but yet be mentally absorbed with thoughts about the topic, thereby preventing him from attending to what is happening in his social world and making him appear aloof and disinterested in others. In addition to potentially interfering with the use of appropriate social skills, in all three of these examples the child with ASD would stand out from peers as a result of the repetitive behavior or restricted interest, often drawing negative attention from peers as a result.

Thought Disturbance

Historically ASD and childhood psychosis have been viewed as largely interchangeable. The absence or near-absence of speech, social skills deficits, odd mannerisms, and unusual interests and beliefs that are often very intense can present very similarly to psychosis. However, research does not indicate increased susceptibility to thought disorders or forms of severe mental illness such as schizophrenia in people with ASD. Although a child with ASD might also have a thought disorder, its occurrence is rare (e.g., Dossetor, 2007). Symptoms of a possible thought disorder warrant thorough evaluation, including taking the family history, before formally diagnosing the patient or initiating specific psychopharmacological or therapeutic treatment. My clinical experience suggests that intense interests can resemble symptoms of a thought disorder (i.e., delusional thinking), especially when the child thinks about the topic of interest almost constantly.

The tendency to perseverate on a topic, combined with unusual speech patterns and difficulty in interpreting the environment, is exemplified in the following case. "Julio," a 13-year-old boy with HFA, had a long-standing intense interest in supernatural matters; he was an avid reader of books on reincarnation and life after death and had an extensive collection of videos on the subject. His parents, who were deeply religious, brought Julio in for treatment because they were concerned that he might be psychotic. He claimed to hear the voice of God, and he would speak at length about how he could tell if someone would have an afterlife after death or if the person was an "evildoer" and therefore would go to hell. Upon being questioned further, Julio explained that if someone lied he or she would not get to an afterlife—that because of the lie, the person was an evildoer. He related this belief to what he had read in a book on religion several months earlier. When he had asked his parents about it, they had agreed that lying was wrong. When asked about the voice he heard, Julio explained that the voice came to him when he felt tempted or really wanted to do something that he knew he shouldn't do—say, like taking an extra cookie after his mother had told him not to. The evaluator believed he was not having an actual auditory hallucination but instead was referring to his internal self-guiding thoughts (e.g., "I shouldn't have another cookie—Mom said no") in an unusual, externally oriented, way. The voice was not constant and seemed to help Julio make appropriate judgments and decisions. In this case, it seemed that Julio presented with behaviors indicative of a possible thought disorder that were more readily explained by his ASD— rigidity in beliefs and rules (lying is wrong, always, and leads to damnation), circumscribed and intense interests (in religion and the afterlife), and tendencies toward literal interpretation (taking a message—perhaps meant metaphorically—from a book and applying it broadly).

Assessment of Social Skills

Decisions on how best to evaluate and monitor a child's skill deficits and progress are both difficult and critical. A thoroughgoing evaluation prior to starting the intervention and sensitive ongoing monitoring of the treatment's progress will guide the delivery process and inform the clinician by answering these key questions:

- What are the specific skills the child most needs to learn or practice?
- How successful is the intervention?
- Is it time to "switch gears" and try something new?

There are multiple approaches and tools available for assessing social skills and social skills deficits but no consensus on a single "best approach" for youths with ASD. Following are some of the more common types of measures one might consider.

Observational Data

A child's use of socially appropriate (or inappropriate) skills can be assessed through observational measures. These observational approaches can be either highly structured and formal (e.g., coding specific behaviors in predetermined time intervals) or quite informal (e.g., qualitative data on how the child behaves with peers during lunch). One method of observational evaluation is "functional assessment" (Iwata, Dorsey, Slifer, Bauman, & Richman, 1982). Based on operant learning theory, functional assessment seeks to identify which specific variables either contribute to a target behavior or prevent a positive behavior, such as initiation with peers, from occurring. This approach to assessment can be particularly useful in school settings.

Consider the following example. A teacher asks the school psychologist to conduct a functional assessment of a student in her class because she wants to understand why the student makes loud animal sounds (e.g., mooing like a cow) that disrupt the other students and bring him unwanted attention and teasing. The psychologist conducts two 30-minute observations of the student on separate days. She records the number of times he engages in the target behavior (making animal sounds) to get a baseline frequency and collects additional data on what happens right before the target behavior (e.g., the student is watching other students in the class) and what happens immediately afterward (e.g., the teacher asks him to stop, and his peers laugh). Based on the antecedents and consequences of the behavior, the psychologist develops a hypothesis about the target behavior. In this example, she hypothesizes that the student is making sounds to get the teacher's and his peers' attention.

To test this hypothesis, the school psychologist manipulates the variables of interest and observes whether there is any effect on the targeted behavior. In this situation, she asks that the teacher give lots of attention to the student when he is seated quietly doing his work and ignore him whenever he starts to make sounds. This example depicts an intervention based on the principle of differential reinforcement of other behavior (DRO). Once the variables associated with the targeted behavior have been identified and the intervention based on the hypotheses drawn from the functional assessment has been completed (i.e., the teacher gives differential reinforcement/attention to the student), follow-up observation determines whether the intervention was successful in reducing the inappropriate behavior. If the behavior persists, further observation and intervention follow. In Figure 2.1, we can see how data gathered from observations during implementation of a DRO intervention might appear in graphical form. The number of inappropriate vocalizations during a particular class period (e.g., math) are recorded. The first phase (baseline) shows the total number of inappropriate vocalizations made daily in math class during the week before implementation of the differential reinforcement, followed by the intervention (week 2), then the pattern of vocalizations following withdrawal of the intervention (week 3). As the data are depicted, the inappropriate noises decreased after the

progress based on his or her observations of the client's behavior. So much is invested in improvement that the practitioner is apt to "see" more improvement than a more objective observer would likely see.

In addition to reducing biased observations by employing third-party observers, it is important that the observations be carried out as unobtrusively as possible. This requirement might necessitate that the person conducting the assessment observe from behind a one-way mirror or from another room—or at the very least observe interactions from the periphery and allow enough time for the subject child/adolescent to acclimate to the presence of the rater. To collect usable valid baseline data against which to determine whether real change has occurred, the observed behaviors must be stable. Otherwise, it is impossible to determine whether the change is attributable to the treatment or to something else, such as the novelty of the observer's presence.

The field of applied behavior analysis has a long history of using functional analytic approaches for children who have ASD. For further information on this approach and how to conduct such an assessment, the reader is referred to Hanley, Iwata, and McCord (2003). An example of a less structured, modified functional assessment that can be done with the parents and the child with ASD is provided in the Appendix in Form 1. This handout can be completed during the initial treatment sessions and subsequently used to guide the choice of intervention(s). The therapist gathers information about the social concerns (the client's behavior), as well as the antecedents and consequences, in as much detail as possible. I find that it is usually most helpful to fill out this form with both the parent(s) and child present, to get both perspectives. Once the family understands the process of carefully observing and collecting relevant data, I often assign further functional assessments as homework for both the parents and child to do between sessions. Figure 2.2 is a sample functional assessment form completed for 14-year-old "Justin." The first entry is by his mother and the second by Justin. Both behaviors recorded involve verbal aggression, likely related to Justin's stress or anxiety about school.

Rating Scales

Paper-and-pencil rating scales are useful because they can be completed quickly, usually in less than 15 minutes, and provide a basis upon which to compare a child's social skills functioning to that of other children. Typically, the measure is completed by someone who knows the child well, such as her parent or teacher.

Perhaps the most frequently used parent report quantitative measure of social skills is the Social Skills Rating System (SSRS; Gresham &

Date and time	Child's behavior (Described in observable, measurable terms)	Antecedent (What was happening right beforehand?)	Consequence (What followed, including parent/sibling reactions?)	Any effects on family functioning? (Your thoughts on what caused or maintained the anxiety)
Dec. 7 (Friday) 3:30 P.M.	Justin yelled at his little brother, went to bedroom and slammed door.	Got off school bus and came inside the house. I asked him to change his clothes and put his things away.	We left Justin alone for about an hour, then I went to his room to talk to him.	It upsets his little brother, puts a strain on the whole family. I get angry and am worried about him. Hypothesis: Justin feels so stressed after being at school all day that he needs time to decompress by himself.
Dec. 10 (Monday) 7:00 A.M.	I told my mom off (yelled, swore), then walked away while she was talking to me.	She told me to get dressed for school— that I was going to be late for school.	Nothing—I still had to go to school. But my mom got upset with me, and I felt bad about yelling at her.	Mom got mad, I felt bad. Hypothesis: I knew the bus was coming and don't need her reminding me.

FIGURE 2.2. Functional assessment of social skills deficits for Justin.

36

Elliott, 1990). The SSRS was developed to help screen for social behavior difficulties in typically developing children. Although not created for use with children on the autism spectrum, the SSRS has been used extensively in research studies to evaluate skills change. Its ability to detect treatment progress in youths on the spectrum has not been firmly established, however (White et al., 2007). The Social Responsiveness Scale (SRS; Constantino & Gruber, 2005) is a commercially available rating scale specifically designed for use with children who have ASD. The SRS provides a dimensional measure of severity of social deficits that can be used for screening purposes. In addition to the global functioning index, the SRS has five treatment subscales designed to evaluate change as a function of treatment. A second ASD-specific measure is the Autism Social Skills Profile (ASSP; Bellini & Hopf, 2007), which focuses exclusively on the child's present level of social functioning (i.e., not other ASD core symptoms, such as repetitive behaviors). The ASSP may be useful in treatment planning and providing information on deficits specific to autism. It is not yet commercially available, although preliminary research on its use is promising (Bellini & Hopf, 2007).

There are no clear recommendations on the "best" rating scale for assessing the degree of the client's social deficit and then tracking change during treatment. Although the SRS, for instance, has been used with some success in treatment outcome research (White, Koenig, & Scahill, 2010), it is not as widely recognized or known as the SSRS. Clinicians can use whichever measure they feel most comfortable with, but they may want to consider using a secondary scale if the results prove to be not consistent with other indices of change, such as parental observational data or anecdotal reports.

Interviews

There is currently no commercially available structured interview specifically designed to assess the social functioning in people with ASD. However, a semistructured clinical interview can be useful in evaluating social skills growth. In clinical settings this interview may constitute the primary assessment conducted at the beginning of treatment. Interviewing the child provides valuable information on how the child presents to someone relatively unfamiliar with him or her, but the primary drawback is that it does not provide detailed firsthand information on the child's interactions with peers. A parent interview is useful in gathering data on the child's social history, including problems at school and what friendships the child has had. Interviews are probably most useful for gathering data to inform the treatment rather than for objectively evaluating change during the treatment. Throughout treatment, of course, both the parent and child should be asked about their impressions of the therapy and how they think things are progressing. Form 2 in the Appendix is a very brief Social History Interview that can be used with the client and parent. Depending on the client's main referral concern, more information would need to be gathered on that particular subject.

Qualitative and Sociometric Data

Qualitative descriptive information on the child's social status can be used to supplement the interview to inform the intervention ultimately selected. To gather sociometric data, the clinician might ask the teacher how well liked the child is or if she has a best friend in class. Information on how the child is received by peers and her social status (e.g., neglected, rejected) can inform treatment goals. Other information that can be useful include the frequency of playdates or how often the child gets together with friends outside of school. Note, however, that playdates arranged and coordinated by parents are much different than outings that the child initiates. Formal sociometric ratings, such as peer rankings of social status, are time consuming and typically reserved for research purposes. However, gathering information on the child's day-to-day social experiences with peers and the quantity and quality of peer friendships provides a relatively straightforward real-world index of social functioning.

In addition to data on social status, information on the acceptability of the intervention should be gathered from both parent and child. If the family/parent/child does not agree with the intervention approach taken or doesn't believe that the child is capable of doing what the therapist asks, improvement in social skills will not occur. It is imperative that the client and parents be "on the same page" with the therapist and have some confidence in the ability of the helper. In my own experience, this bond is critical to establish at the outset of treatment, especially for school-age children and adolescents because they have often been the recipient of other programs in the past through school and/or community-based clinicians. I like to ask what they have tried in the past, how things went, what they liked or didn't like, and what they might hope will be different this time. Despite these personal preferences, the extent to which a child or parent likes the intervention does not necessarily correlate with observed and actual gains in social skills (e.g., Provencal, 2003).

These four types of assessments—observational tools, rating scales, interviews, and qualitative/sociometric data and tools—in respect to four attributes—namely, structure, data quality, bias, and time—are depicted in Figure 2.3. These ratings are based on my own clinical and

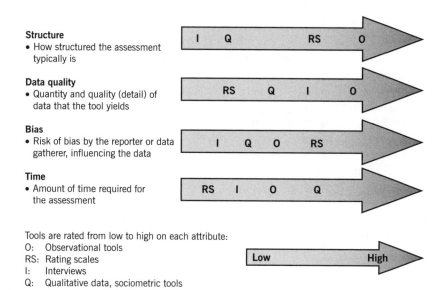

Structure
• How structured the assessment typically is

| I   Q   RS   O |

Data quality
• Quantity and quality (detail) of data that the tool yields

| RS   Q   I   O |

Bias
• Risk of bias by the reporter or data gatherer, influencing the data

| I   Q   O   RS |

Time
• Amount of time required for the assessment

| RS   I   O   Q |

Tools are rated from low to high on each attribute:
O: Observational tools
RS: Rating scales
I: Interviews
Q: Qualitative data, sociometric tools

| Low   High |

FIGURE 2.3. Attributes of different types of social skills assessment tools.

research experience with the tools and therefore are fairly subjective. Each type of tool is rated on the four attributes relative to the other tools; they are ordinal, not interval, rankings. Of course, there is considerable variability within each type of tool. Some interviews, for example, are very structured, although most clinical intake interviews are not standardized. Likewise, asking about the frequency of playdates (a form of qualitative data collection) will take considerably less time than a more formalized assessment of the child's social status in the classroom.

Deciding which measure(s) to use for a given situation or client can be challenging. In choosing a battery of measures to use, consider the following suggestions:

- Use multiple informants. Whenever possible, a child's social skills should be assessed by using more than one informant—such as both the teacher and the parent(s).
- Use several measurement tools. Multiple modalities of assessment (e.g., both rating scales *and* interviews) will usually be superior to relying on only one type of measurement tool.
- Collect information across diverse settings. Children with ASD struggle with skill generalization, that is, applying a skill learned in one situation (e.g., therapy) to other situations (school, home,

etc.). Therefore, the clinician is well advised to get rating scales and interview data from both the parent and the child's homeroom teacher, to better understand how the child acts at school *and* at home.

Based on the data gathered about the nature of the client's social deficits, a case conceptualization is developed that is used to guide intervention and monitoring during treatment. One possible format for such a conceptualization is given in Figure 2.4 (a blank version is provided in the Appendix, Form 3). This case conceptualization may be used as a template to be modified as needed, depending on the context of the intervention (e.g., school, clinic) and the particular format (e.g., group or individual counseling). I like to share the case conceptualization with the parents and usually with the child, too, to ensure that we have a shared vision of both the treatment and the agreed-upon treatment goals.

Case Example

"Maria" has always been interested in the weather. In early adolescence, this interest became the source of great anxiety. Following a severe thunderstorm when Maria was home alone, she became intensely frightened of thunderstorms and windstorms. Afterward, she began watching the weather channel every day and studying weather patterns. She feared a big storm and had great difficulty in controlling her worries about it. Her anxiety interfered with her family relationships and even led to her avoidance of social activities.

She frequently asked for reassurance from her parents about the weather, refused to leave the house when bad weather was even a possibility, and begged her parents to come home early from work if a storm was predicted. Although Maria never had very many friends, she did have two relatively close girlfriends from her church. Once, while with her friends, she had become inconsolably upset during a lightning storm. Maria was certain that the girls remembered the incident and judged her harshly as a consequence. She therefore subsequently refused to spend time with them, despite their entreaties and offers to get together afterward. Maria's fears and her general embarrassment owing to these fears severely limited her ability to engage in age-appropriate social relationships, thereby leaving her parents exasperated.

Maria's parents eventually referred her for individual therapy when her fears failed to abate on their own despite the parents' repeated reassurances. In addition to a primary diagnosis of PDD-NOS, which was previously diagnosed, Maria met the criteria for a specific phobia, natu-

Name: JB	Diagnoses (based on all available data):
Parent(s): Ms. B	Axis I PDD-NOS (ASD)
Age: 15	Axis II None
Contact Information:	Axis III None
12A McArthur Street	Axis IV academic difficulty, recent of cousin
Anytown, VA 12345	Axis V 64
PDD-NOS (ASD)	

Social Skills Concerns (in order, from most severe; based on observation, clinical interview, other assessments):	Primary Social Skills Deficits (parent report):
1. gets frustrated when peers don't see things her way	1. talks over other people
2. monologue speech—irritates other people	2. does not pick up on people's cues about conversations, especially when to end
3. lack of flexibility about rules at school	Primary Social Skills Deficits (child report):
4. socially isolated, lonely	1. no friends, no one to sit with at lunch
	2. people at school don't follow the rules, I get bothered

Selected Social Skills Target(s) (one or two, to be targeted initially in treatment):

Improve social flexibility (accepting others when they don't follow rules); Improve conversational turn-taking

Hypotheses about Causal and Maintaining Factors (observations, parent reports, assessment results):

J tends to engage in black-or-white thinking (e.g., "my way is the only right way—others are wrong") and has some very intense interests, which she enjoys talking about. She also has only limited opportunities in her daily life to practice new skills with peers.

Intervention Strategies:

Cognitive–behavioral therapy—cognitive restructuring, improve flexibility skills, practice conversational skills (esp. turn-taking, listening), relaxation strategies (e.g., self-talk) to manage frustration

Monitoring Plan (methods of assessment to be used and frequency of assessment):

SRS (pre-, midpoint, endpoint), parent and child interview, clinical observation, teacher report (over telephone)

| Strengths/Interests of Client: | Potential Barriers to Treatment and Solutions: |
| Intelligent, motivated to make friends, supportive family | Very high standards for herself, rigid, still mourning cousin (with family) (practice imperfection with homework assignments, grief counseling for family) |

FIGURE 2.4. Case conceptualization.

ral environment type. Maria's psychologist provided education to Maria and her parents about PDD-NOS and the extent of her anxiety problems; they discussed how her anxiety affected her relationships with family and friends; and they agreed to engage in cognitive-behavioral therapy, including exposure. Exposure therapy was conducted to address the phobia, and her parents were asked to support Maria's efforts to cope but not to provide reassurance in response to her repetitive questioning when anxious, as this response only temporarily served to reduce her anxiety. Cognitive-behavioral treatment addressed Maria's beliefs and assumptions about her friends and their thoughts about her. Maria accepted that they probably did not care, or perhaps even remember, that she had gotten so upset during a storm. Ultimately, Maria's anxiety eventually diminished enough that she began socializing more often with her friends.

CHAPTER 3

Types of Interventions and Adaptations for ASD

Social skills training is neither a novel intervention nor a unique treatment for ASD. Practitioners and educators have been developing and implementing programs to try to improve the social skills of children and adolescents for decades. However, when intervening with youths who have autism and related conditions, certain adaptations can help make intervention more effective. This chapter provides a broad overview of the various types of intervention and some of the primary modifications, or adaptations, generally helpful in working with students who have ASD. Later chapters go into greater depth on specific interventions and strategies. The suggestions provided in this chapter are broad in nature and are based on what is "typically" helpful for people with ASD. In developing a treatment regimen for a specific child, consideration must be given to that child's learning style, any possible processing deficits, and other clinical concerns.

Types of Interventions

In a qualitative review of studies on social skills programming for young children with ASD, McConnell (2002) divided interventions into five broad categories: (1) environmental modifications; (2) child-specific interventions; (3) collateral skills interventions; (4) peer-mediated programs; and (5) comprehensive programs. Thinking of interventions in terms of these categories can be helpful in planning treatment for a given child or group of students. See Table 3.1 for specific examples of interventions falling into each of these categories. Most of the examples provided in Table 3.1 apply to educational settings. The listed "pros"

TABLE 3.1. Five Types of Interventions: Benefits, Drawbacks, and Examples

Intervention type	Benefits	Drawbacks	Examples
Environmental modifications	May promote social interaction naturally, often by proximity to peers	Often not substantive as a stand-alone intervention	• Arranging classroom desks into "clusters" with the subject child seated near socially skilled and friendly peers • Making classroom transitions (e.g., from one topic to the next) predictable
Child-specific interventions	Often necessary to teach requisite skills, especially for skill acquisition deficits	Limited generalization of skill use; integrating peers into intervention can help	• Prompts (reminders) are provided by an adult to initiate with peers • School counselor meets with the child at the end of each day to review targeted social skills, providing reinforcement for social initiations the student made during the day
Collateral skills interventions	Can be easily integrated into child's natural environment, school contexts	Without explicit help on the requisite skills (e.g., working with peers in a group), the child may struggle	• Creating a classwide play (drama) in which each student plays a role • Organizing a small-group collaborative academic project (e.g., class presentations on video games)
Peer-mediated programs	Prompting or feedback from a peer may be more powerful or meaningful than that coming from adult	May make the peer feel obligated and may "identify" or disclose the child with ASD to others	• Socially skilled peer is identified and taught how to encourage verbal communication with his or her ASD peer • An after-school social group with same-age peers is organized around the shared interests of the children (e.g., marine biology)
Comprehensive programs	May be more effective than a single intervention approach	If helpful, it is difficult to determine why, that is, which aspects of intervention are crucial; also may be more time-consuming to plan	• Integrating direct social skills instruction (that is child-specific) with peer coaching (peer-mediated) • Classwide daily social skills instruction followed by "free time" for work on group projects

(benefits) and "cons" (drawbacks) are based on available research as well as firsthand experience.

Environmental modifications typically refer to changes made to the child's classroom or other environment that are expected to promote improved social functioning. Examples include arranging the seating in a classroom so that any child with ASD is deliberately placed near socially skilled peers or, in addition, posting visual reminders around the classroom that encourage students to engage in practicing targeted social skills. Interventions that are designated as child-specific involve direct one-on-one instruction and generally focus on the specific skill deficits of each child. Collateral skills interventions, in contrast, do not teach specific social skills directly but instead emphasize related skills (e.g., language development) that in turn promote social development. Peer-mediated programs seek to involve one's peers in facilitating (via teaching, modeling, reinforcement, etc.) social skills use among children with ASD. Finally, comprehensive intervention programs integrate multiple teaching approaches simultaneously (e.g., direct instruction and language development) to maximally useful effect.

Typically, utilizing more than one type of approach proves helpful. An elementary school student, for instance, may have specific environmental modifications built into his individualized education plan (IEP) to address particular social skills concerns and, additionally, be assigned a peer buddy for less structured times (e.g., physical education class) at school. He might also concurrently receive individual social skills training from the school counselor.

"Emory," a fourth grader, enjoyed being around his peers, but would quickly become overwhelmed and agitated with too much social or academic stimulation. In his IEP, Emory was provided certain in-school accommodations—specifically, keyboard aids for written assignments and abbreviated versions of most in-class assignments—owing to his struggle with handwriting and because of his slow pace in completing work. These various problems contributed to a heightened sense of anxiety and anger, which in turn inhibited his ability to interact socially with classmates. In physical education and study hall (free time), he worked alongside a preselected peer who was both socially skilled and well aware of Emory's limitations. The peer made sure that Emory had a place to sit with the other children and also modeled appropriate peer interaction skills. In class, the teacher reminded the peer buddy about ways to help Emory and made sure he interacted appropriately with him. Twice a week, Emory received 30 minutes of direct social skills instruction from the school counselor before school. Emory's case demonstrates integration of three separate approaches to intervention—environmental, peer-mediated, and child-specific. The modality of intervention can also vary—that is, the training can be done one-on-one (therapist and child), in a group format (with two or more children at a time), or systemically (e.g., classwide).

Adaptations to Interventions for ASD

Regardless of the type of intervention chosen, certain practices promote better social skills acquisition and improved skills performance by youths with ASD, including the following (which are explored in greater detail below):

- A high level of structure and routine
- An adequate "dosage" of the intervention
- A safe, nurturing environment
- The involvement of peers
- Matching skills training to the child's deficit areas
- The use of a natural environment

Structure

Youths with ASD thrive on consistency and predictability. For a person on the autism spectrum, knowing what to expect can allay behavioral problems that could impede the progress of the intervention. In fact, *not knowing what to expect or how to act* may lead to anxiety that limits the child's ability to fully participate in the learning process, thereby short-circuiting the potential success of the intervention. Providing a clear structure for the child, regardless of the intervention implemented, is helpful (e.g., White et al., 2007). Structure refers to consistency across training sessions (therapy visits, etc.), the routine within each training session, and predictability for the child. One simple way to instill structure is for the therapist to follow the same, preset agenda for each session. A session might include the following components, in order: welcome and warm-up, homework review, work on the current skill or exercise, assignment for the week, and time to talk about the child's topic of choice. Figure 3.1 presents a sample (generalized) session agenda. I usually post (or write on the whiteboard) the specific agenda at the start of each session as a reminder to the child. For younger children, the agenda might be accompanied by images or pictures. For older children, I often have them write out the agenda.

Another consideration in imposing predictability is to have the rules for the therapy made explicit from the very outset. The content of the

---

1. Welcome

a. Brief time for "small talk," greetings

2. Review

a. Discuss content and skills covered in the preceding session

b. Discuss homework assigned, and complete it now if not accomplished between the sessions

3. New Learning

a. Teach skill(s)

b. Practice skill(s) during the session

4. Assignment

a. Assign homework or practice exercises for the coming week

b. Identify how the client will record his or her homework (e.g., any written worksheets?)

5. Free time

a. Brief time (e.g., 5 minutes) for the child to select a preferred topic of conversation, such as a special interest or something happening at school

6. Wrap-Up and Parental Feedback

a. Bring parent(s) in to summarize the session's content

b. Let parent(s) know what homework was assigned and request their feedback

c. Good-byes

FIGURE 3.1. Sample session agenda.

rules depends on the context of the intervention and the child. In individual therapy, for instance, the rules might address expectations for timeliness and attendance, assignment completion, participation and honesty, and behavior during the session (e.g., no obscene language, respect for personal space). Most children appreciate the boundaries and expectations that fair and clearly identified rules impart. This observation is especially true of children with ASD. At the start of treatment, I tell the new client that I have certain rules for our time together such as mutual respect for each other and being prepared and on time for every session. Depending on the client and what information I have about him or her in advance, I might add to or change my rules. For example, one child I treated had great difficulty leaving the toys and playing cards available in the lobby behind when it was time for his session to start. I recalled this particular circumstance from his initial evaluation. In his case I therefore created the rule that he could bring one toy from the lobby into the session but that he had to set it on the bookshelf until the final 5 minutes of the session, when we would play with the object together. Encourage the child to suggest any rules he or she would like observed, as well. Asking for the child's input demonstrates the therapist's respect for the child and a sincere desire to know the child's preferences. Some degree of predictability and structure can be achieved in every type of intervention and whatever modality, whether individual therapy sessions, group practices, or time spent with peer mentors.

"Dosage"

The severity and pervasiveness of social deficits in ASD necessitate that the training experience be highly intensive. Thus, the "dosage" of treatment is typically much stronger than that in social skills development interventions for other clinical populations. A doctor would hardly expect a 2-month trial of insulin to be sufficient for the treatment of a patient with Type I diabetes. Similarly, a time-limited social skills training intervention cannot be expected to dramatically improve social functioning in a lasting way for a person with ASD. Brief interventions, even when intensive, will almost always need to be fortified with some type of ancillary support. The child's parents, for instance, should ideally be trained alongside the child who is in individual therapy so that they can promote his or her skills use in the home and community. In general, the therapist involves the parent(s) in every treatment session, usually at the end, to review what skill was covered and identify strategies that can be tried at home to continue to practice the skill. The therapist might then directly observe as the parent helps his or her child practice the new skill. The therapist could thereby provide immediate feedback to the parent and the child and make modifications to the training if needed (e.g., remind the parent to praise attempted target behavior, even when not perfect). Another helpful option is to give prepared handouts to the parent summarizing the skill(s) covered during the session and suggesting how the child can best practice the skill at home during the week. My colleague Kathleen Koenig, of the Yale Child Study Center, and I used parent letters to describe the skills we taught during a social skills training program for school-age children with ASD. Three sample parent letters, summarizing the skills taught during the sessions, are provided in Figures 3.2–3.4. The first two are from social skills training groups, and the third is from an individual (client–therapist) session.

Dear Parents,

    This week in our social skills group we will be focusing on conversational turn-taking. The group coleader, Jay, and I will also continue to observe the children's behavior during the group session to get a better understanding of each child's social strengths and areas in which he or she can improve.

    In today's session, after our welcome activity and review of the group's rules (staying still, mouth quiet, hands to self, eyes on speaker), we will play a game involving turn-taking in a conversation. The objective of this activity is to practice starting conversations with peers and making appropriate and contingent (i.e., on-topic) responses/questions during conversations. We work in teams of two, with the other players watching each team practice. As the two players build their conversation, they earn more points in the game. If they lose the thread of the conversation or get too off-topic, then a new team gets to try.

    During the coming week, to practice the skills of turn-taking in conversation and staying on topic, consider adapting one of your child's favorite games (e.g., checkers, chess) so that with each turn each player has to say something related to the topic. With each new game, a new topic can be chosen. If your child enjoys friendly competition, you could even keep a tally of the number of on-topic responses made during each game.

    We hope everyone is enjoying the group so far. Please contact us if you have any questions or suggestions!

                                 Sincerely,

FIGURE 3.2. Parent letter: Sample 1.

Dear Parents,

    As in last week's group session, we will first do
a welcome activity (talking about what we are looking
forward to this weekend, and one thing we've learned
about someone else in the group over the past 2 weeks)
and review the group's rules (staying still, mouth quiet,
hands to self, eyes on speaker).
    There are two main activities during today's group
session. The first activity is called Conversation Ball.
This game is played by the whole group—we toss a ball back
and forth among players, and with each toss the person
throwing the ball must make a comment or ask a question
that is related to the preceding comment or question. The
learning objective of this game is to practice initiating
and maintaining a conversation. Each child gets an
opportunity to start a new game, or conversation, with
a topic of his or her choosing. The second activity is
Telephone Tag. Our version of the classic game involves
each person sequentially whispering a brief message or
story to the next person until the message gets to the
last person in the circle. The last person then tells the
story that he or she heard out loud. This game provides
the kids the opportunity to practice multiple conversation
skills, including listening carefully to what another
person is saying (to understand the message), controlling
voice volume (one must whisper to prevent the other kids
from hearing the story), and turn-taking. It is also a fun
way to get the point across that what one person "hears"
is not always what was "intended."
    During the week, to practice conversational skills
(e.g., turn-taking, voice volume, staying on topic),
consider playing Conversation Ball as a family game. You
and your child can play alone or bring in other family
members. Point out all the things that he or she is doing
right (e.g., "I really like how quietly you said that!"),
and prompt him or her about the things to continue to work
on.

            Sincerely,

            _____

FIGURE 3.3. Parent letter: Sample 2.

Dear Parent,

    We have been working for the past few weeks on appreciating Tom's social strengths and his particular areas of difficulty. He seems to have an appreciation for the things that are more challenging for him, like greeting others in a friendly, approachable way and accurately interpreting other people's nonverbal behaviors and emotional states. In our session today, we talked about identifying emotions in other people and labeling them. We looked at pictures in magazines together and discussed the emotions expressed by the models and what cues indicated that particular emotion (e.g., "His arms are folded and he is scowling, so he must be angry"). We also read some hypothetical vignettes (stories) together (e.g., "Jake just got his test back in math class. He thought he had done really well, but instead he got a D-. How do you think Jake feels?"). Tom tried to identify the emotions of the character and then act out whatever emotion he thought might be most appropriate. Afterward, I acted out the emotions, and Tom was to respond appropriately—for instance, by offering a kind word or a smile.

    If you'd like to continue to work on helping Tom accurately identify and respond to other people's emotions, one suggestion is to look at books and magazines with him—something similar to what we did today in the session. Or you can do this activity while watching a movie or TV show. Point out pictures (scenes from a show) that depict strong emotions, and start a dialogue with him about what the person might be feeling (e.g., "his forehead is all wrinkly, and he is shaking his finger—he must be angry")—or consider scenes showing multiple people, and comment on the characters' relative standing and personal closeness or distance from one another.

    As always, please let me know if you have any suggestions or questions.

                      Sincerely,

FIGURE 3.4. Parent letter: Sample 3.

Other examples of ways that targeted intervention can be further fortified include a time-limited social skills group intervention followed by several "booster" sessions (e.g., to review skills every 2–4 weeks) or a follow-up ongoing group that meets regularly. In other words, a single dose of treatment, such as a semester-long after-school group, is typically not enough reinforcement. *Children with ASD need ongoing training and support to improve social functioning.* In addition, improvement will be more likely if more than one type of intervention is applied. In sum, both *duration* and *intensity* must be considered.

Safety

Many people with ASD have been teased, bullied, or even physically assaulted because of their perceived immature, inappropriate, or awkward behaviors and poorly developed social skills. Thus, the importance that an atmosphere of acceptance and nurturing plays within any social skills intervention cannot be readily overstated. Especially for older children and teenagers starting a group-based intervention for the first time with similar-age peers, developing an environment that provides support and caring among group members and leaders is critically important. In my own experience, many teenagers are apprehensive about interacting with peers, and they carry a great deal of emotional "baggage" owing to their past negative social experiences. As discussed in greater detail in Chapter 4 on group-based interventions, soliciting group members' input about how they wish to be treated and their preferred rules of behavior (e.g., regarding respect and confidentiality) is absolutely imperative.

Peer Involvement

There is growing acknowledgment within the scientific community of the key importance of peer involvement in social skills interventions (e.g., Barry et al., 2003; Rogers, 2000). No matter how well intentioned adults may be about trying to improve an adolescent's social functioning, inevitably they simply cannot relate to teenagers as well as other teenagers do. As I have witnessed countless times, feedback from a peer—especially a peer whom a youth with ASD respects—can often lead to a behavioral change or teach a concept I may have been trying fruitlessly to impart over several previous occasions. The case described at the end of this chapter illustrates quite clearly the massive influence a well-chosen peer tutor can have!

Good peers can be either neurotypical (i.e., not have an ASD) or even other children with spectrum conditions. I have found both types to be very helpful. Peers who have ASD can serve as a good normalizing influence, for example, when the subject realizes that other children experience similar difficulties. Also, the two often do share similar interests and can develop long-lasting friendships that extend beyond the course of the intervention. Typically developing peers without ASD are helpful in modeling age-appropriate skills. They are conversant with the jargon used by the child's peer group and tend to be better versed on events of interest to young people as compared to most adult therapists. For example, while some adolescents with ASD are able to introduce themselves to adults while sounding very much like their neurotypical peers (e.g., "Hello—how are you?"), such a greeting would not be appropriate for how one 16-year-old typically greets another 16-year-old! In other words, neurotypical peers' involvement can offer a needed entrée into the client's peer group that people outside the group simply can't match. Properly educating neurotypical peer tutors about ASD and their role in the intervention (group experience or mentoring system) is important. They should be provided specific information about what to expect, the types of challenges that people with ASD typically have, and what role they are expected to play in the intervention.

Personally, I have found that, while training tutors properly at the start of the intervention is crucial, providing specific instructions before each session (e.g., "Today I want you to sit by Jack and help him initiate") is also helpful and advisable. The rules relating to confidentiality must be expressly discussed and defined before a peer tutor becomes involved in any social skills intervention. Confidentiality must be assured, regardless of the intervention. Tutors need to fully understand that they are not to discuss the group or its interactions with their friends at school and that respect for each participant's privacy is sacrosanct. This requirement is especially critical in smaller isolated towns or rural areas where often there is only one middle school or high school and the likelihood of the group members seeing one another outside of the community is especially high. I normally have all peer tutors as well as the groups' members—as part of the written consent for the intervention—agree to and sign a statement of confidentiality. This statement generally warrants that they agree not to discuss the group, including the other kids in the group or what group members say, with people outside of the group. Of course, they can and should talk about their own experience in the group with their parents as they wish. I again verbally review the rules relating to mutual respect and confidentiality for peers in the group during the first session. Below, in question-and-answer format, is an excerpt from a consent document for peer tutors agreed to by the child that I have used in intervention groups:

Will you tell anyone what I say?
We will not share your specific input/thoughts with your teachers, your parents, or your friends. But we will give your parents a summary of what we worked on in each group meeting. If you were to tell us that someone is hurting you, or that you might hurt yourself or someone else, however, we are required to tell people in authority so they can help you.

Also, it is important that what is said in the groups remain confidential, meaning that you and the other teens in the group should not talk about it with people outside of the group. This includes not telling friends or other people either who is in the group or what is said in the group.

Matching Training Skills to Deficits

As Gresham et al. (2001) have suggested, the child's type of skills deficit should determine specifically which skills are taught and how they are taught (see Chapter 1). Although the concept of matching the training to the skills deficit type is not really unique to therapy for ASD, it often seems to be overlooked. To review briefly, the main types of skills deficits, from the child's point of view, are:

- *Skill acquisition deficit*: "What am I supposed to do?"
- *Performance deficit*: "I know what to do—but when do I do it?"
- *Fluency deficit*: "I am trying to do it, but it's not working!"

A fluency deficit, for example, requires that one focus on practice and generalization rather than on learning why the skill is important. For a child with a fluency deficit in the skill of initiating interactions with peers, for example, if the therapist spends time teaching the skill and explaining why it is an important skill to have, the child will probably feel frustrated and eventually respond emphatically that "I already know that!" A much more useful approach is to observe the child using the skill—videotaping him if possible—and then give feedback on implementing the skill, refining the skill and then repeatedly practicing it to improve fluency. The therapist can usually form accurate impressions about what type(s) of deficits a child has from the intake interview and his or her responses to certain rating scales (see Chapter 2).

Natural Environment

Finally, using a natural environment in which to practice new skills aids in learning and flexibly applying the skills in the child's target environments. In other words, naturalistic practice is important for the generalization of one's skills. The skills should be learned and practiced in situations and environments that approximate as closely as possible those situations and environments in which the child is expected to actually *use* the skills (Bellini & Akullian, 2007; Bellini et al., 2007). Ideally, practice exercises would always occur in the actual place where the problem is encountered, but this arrangement is often not feasible.

In actual practice, a social skills group is normally conducted in a middle school and role plays in a clinic-based group are structured as closely as possible to real-life social situations (e.g., in a cafeteria). In individual therapy, attaining this goal may mean having some skills practice at the child's school. Such practice is usually best conducted after school hours, before trying the skills out during the schoolday with actual peers. A related consideration is that the same skill—say, greeting a person—might look quite different, depending on the environmental context. For example, when calling someone on the phone, the adolescent might learn to say "Hello—it's Jane. Is this a good time to talk?" But in person-to-person contacts, the teen would not use the same skills; instead, she would rely more on nonverbal cues (a smile, eye contact) and say something like, "Hi—how are you?" The specific approach would also vary with the circumstances. When trying to get a store clerk's attention, for instance, one would need to wait until the clerk was free and then approach with a smile to ask for help.

Case Example

"Alan" came to his social skills group every week looking sullen and dejected. He walked to the room where we met with his head down and, once in the room, did not make eye contact with anyone. He kept his arms folded across his chest, slouched down in his chair, and would rarely participate. Alan's behavior affected the overall dynamics of the group, and his demeanor appeared to discourage the participation of others. This type of interaction had been occurring since the start-up of the group 3 weeks earlier. My coleader and I used both direct and indirect approaches to address Alan's behavior. We told him how it looked and how it made us feel worried for him; we tried reflecting his apparent feelings—inquiring about what he must be going through; we developed group activities that we felt confident that Alan would be interested in; and together we viewed videotapes of the group's interactions in the hope that Alan would develop an awareness of how his nonverbal behaviors made others see him as unfriendly, probably resulting in increased disinterest from his peers. It seemed that whatever we tried didn't help in that Alan continued to present as dejected and disinterested.

CHAPTER 4

Social Skills Training Groups

Background on Group-Delivered Interventions

Social skills training groups are very often recommended for people who have autism and related conditions. There is an obvious appeal in choosing group-delivered interventions for facilitating social skills growth in children. The group format affords one the opportunity to practice the new skills in a relatively natural setting. Additionally, being in a group promotes interaction with peers. At the same time, however, youths with ASD typically have great difficulty operating within social groups. As Bauminger (2007) points out, successful group interaction requires a host of relatively high-level skills, such as the ability to attend to multiple auditory signals (i.e., listening skills) and the ability to infer others' intentions and motivations. These skills are normally deficient in children with ASD. Based on a review of the research literature on group-based social skills instruction in ASD (see White et al., 2007), the following conclusions may be drawn:

- Support for group-based instruction is equivocal. While skills gains are reported, they are typically not uniform across participants or skill areas.
- For most children, even with group-based social skills training, there continue to be problems with skills maintenance (the use of skills over time) and generalization (the use of skills in diverse settings).

- It is preferable to have at least some skills practice occur in natural settings.
- Parental involvement in the intervention may help improve outcomes.

Despite the fact that the long-term impact of such interventions on skills growth remains somewhat uncertain, there is strong demand for group-delivered interventions because of the following circumstances: (1) more and more children are being identified with ASD who need services; (2) most social skills curricula are delivered in a group format; and (3) there are obvious benefits to having access to same-age peers with whom to practice in the group. Thus, this ever-increasing demand, combined with a lack of empirically supported curricula to use, leaves clinicians and families in a bind.

My own view is that *social skills groups for youths with ASD can be helpful for some people and in some skills domains.* In my own experience, children who tend to do best in a social skills group are those who have some motivation to improve their skills and make friends, who readily acknowledge that they have some skills deficits that they would like to improve, and who don't exhibit severe maladaptive behaviors that could make interacting with peer group members aversive. But this type of intervention is not a panacea, nor even the best-choice treatment for all kids. If a child has severe anxiety or engages in behaviors that could be unsafe in a group environment (e.g., sudden unprovoked aggression), a group intervention should never be implemented for that child until such behaviors are under control. I inform families fully about both the likely limitations and risks (e.g., the time commitment, the heightened anxiety of being around other kids) and the intended results (namely, improvement in certain skill domains). This type of disclosure is similar to what any practitioner would do during the informed consent process with a client considering any new treatment or medication.

Groups may be offered in a wide variety of settings, such as specialty clinics, schools, and the offices of practitioners who have several clients with similar needs. The group leaders might be psychologists, teachers, occupational therapists, or other helping professionals. The content and focus of skill groups also can vary considerably; groups may address theory of mind, discrete social skills, conversational skills, expanding children's repertoire of interests, building social interest and motivation—the list goes on and on. This chapter reviews promising teaching strategies and more general considerations for running social skills training groups for youths with ASD, based on previous clinical studies, literature reviews, the learning characteristics of people with ASD, and clinical experience. At the close of the chapter, some clinical issues that my colleagues and I have faced in running such groups are briefly addressed.

Content and Strategies

Summarized in Table 4.1 are various strategies that are considered "promising" based on a comprehensive review of the literature on group-based social skills training research (White et al., 2007). These strategies are organized into broad categories that are discussed in greater detail below, along with specific examples. In the section on Further Reading at the end of the book, some currently available curricula developed for

TABLE 4.1. Promising Teaching Strategies for Social Skills Training in ASD

Increase social motivation and esteem

- Start with easily learned skills, gradually intersperse more challenging skills.
- Make teaching fun and predictable—incorporate visuals and set an agenda.
- Incorporate aspects of pivotal response training.

Focus on skills development

- Reduce interfering behaviors.
- Teach age-appropriate lingo and metaphors, address literal interpretations.
- Cover basic social rules (e.g., staying one arm's length away).

Increase social initiations/responses

- Use natural reinforcers for social initiations.
- Reward attempts (shaping).
- Teach and model "age-appropriate" initiations.
- Teach simple social "scripts" for common situations.

Reduce interfering behaviors

- Make rules clear from the outset; use behavior charts.
- Differentially reinforce positive behaviors.
- Conduct functional analysis of interfering behaviors to identify maintenance factors.

Promote skills generalization

- Orchestrate peer involvement.
- Use multiple trainers (parents, siblings) with whom the child can practice skills.
- Be creative: practice in safe natural settings.
- Use time between sessions to practice (homework).

Note. Adapted from White, Koenig, and Scahill (2007, p. 1864) with kind permission from Springer Science + Business Media.

teaching appropriate social skills to youths with ASD are listed. These curricula can be applied in a group format.

Increase Social Motivation and Esteem

More often than not, in the groups I have conducted or observed, the participants exhibit a great deal of anxiety initially, especially during the earliest sessions. For most kids, the group is a novel social experience that occurs in a context that has usually been difficult for them to contend with in the past (i.e., a setting that includes many peers) and that focuses on skill sets that, for them, are problematic. Taken together, it is little wonder that many children are not entirely sure they even want to have anything to do with a social skills group! Fortunately, there are several things the group leaders can do to allay anxieties, increase motivation and help to build self-esteem among group members.

One of the most obvious yet powerful strategies is to *go slow* with teaching. Present lots of opportunities for success, right from the start. It is always preferable, for instance, to make the first group meeting very low-stress and fun. One basic skill might be addressed during the first group meeting, such as learning one another's names, but the main purposes are usually to introduce everyone and build interest in coming to the sessions. Also, as Koegel, Koegel, and Brookman (2005) have emphasized in their work on pivotal response training (PRT), allowing the group members to help choose activities helps to develop their motivation. Leaders should always get input throughout the course of the therapy on the participants' preferences for games, activities, and even snacks. *Older children and adolescents especially want to know that they have a voice in the group and a voice in how it is run.*

Following is a typical agenda that my colleagues and I normally follow during the initial meeting of a new group. We first orient everyone to the agenda, which is posted on a whiteboard or easel so that everyone can see it. We review the time that the group meets and the intended length of the therapy, and also the groups' purpose, saying something like:

> "As we've discussed with each of you individually earlier, this group is *for you*. We are here to figure out better ways for you to make friends and keep friends and, in general, to get along better with people."

This message can be made simpler or more complex based on the needs and ages of the group's participants. Next, I proceed to the introductions. While seated in a circle, we usually start with the group leaders, followed by the typically developing peer tutors, and then go around in turn to the other members. The introductions can be as simple as having each person state his or her name and something about him- or herself (e.g., a hobby, a favorite food). With groups made up of older children, I like to make this exercise into a memory game to help them really focus on learning one another's names while also having fun. In that case, after the first round of introductions, for example, each person might reintroduce the person seated to the left by giving that person's name and one thing he or she learned about that person (e.g., "This is Mike. He goes to Auburn Middle School and likes to eat pizza").

After establishing the group's rules, briefly reviewing confidentiality requirements and the format of the group, and having a snack, we then discuss what specific kinds of skills the kids think they would like to focus on. This discussion can be really helpful to the group leaders in planning curriculum and often the members have pretty good ideas about what exactly they struggle with. Having the participants identify their own skill deficits helps to normalize the social difficulties experienced in the group and to create an atmosphere of helping—it makes maximum feedback "okay." When peer tutors are in the group, they too identify at least one skill to work on improving. As a group leader, I sometimes model this dialogue (e.g., "One thing I know I struggle with is letting other people have a chance to talk. Sometimes I get excited about something and talk too much—so, I'd like to improve that. In fact, if you notice I am talking too much, I would like you to let me know"). In addition, during the snack break the group leaders can poll members about what types of snacks they'd like in the future and what types of games they'd like to play. As just noted, having a say in such matters increases motivation and it also helps everyone get to know one another better. Before finishing the first session, we always play a fun game.

Therapists considering starting a social skills group for youths with ASD often wonder about how to introduce the non-ASD peer tutors to the group. Personally, I tend to not introduce the peer tutor, as such, in a formal sense during the session. However, all of the group members are informed before starting the program that the group will have members with ASD diagnoses and members without ASD who are there to learn skills and help the other people in the group. I have not found it helpful to disclose or discuss diagnostic labels in the context of the therapy for two reasons. First, it is difficult to identify the peer tutor(s) as such without opening up a discussion of diagnoses for the other group members, and it is never my intent to "out" a particular child's diagnosis to the peers—that is his or her decision. Second, and more relevant to the purposes of the intervention, most of the skills addressed (e.g., meeting new peers, talking to members of the opposite sex) within the therapy are skills that most children and teenagers could use help and support with—regardless of the ASD. As is further elaborated in Chapter 6, I have found psychoeducation relating to a client's particular diagnosis to be more logically a component of individual rather than group therapy. I should note, however, that often a discussion about ASD and diagnosis is begun by the group members themselves. When that happens, it can be an incredibly valuable teaching moment. Skills related to self-disclosure, asking sensitive questions tactfully, and honesty become the focus of the discussion. Sometimes a member of the group asks me about another child's diagnosis or whether the other child is a peer tutor. I prefer not to disclose the information myself but instead tell the person inquiring to pose the question directly to the child. Before giving such a suggestion, it is, of course, advisable to talk with group members and do some role play or other training on how to appropriately respond to questions like this and not disclose more than what one is comfortable with.

One game that I have found that works well is to toss around a balloon or a soft ball, the main object being to remember one another's names. In the first round of the game, the rule is that before you toss the ball to anyone you have to say the other person's name first. During the second round, the focus shifts to names *and* eye contact—that is, "Now you have to make sure you make eye contact *and* say the other person's name before throwing the ball." At the end of the group session, I summarize what was taught and discussed, remind participants of when the next group session is scheduled, and always say good-bye.

Focus on Skills Development

Focusing on skills development might seem obvious but in fact can be quite difficult, especially when one is faced with a seemingly endless array of behaviors that are *unwanted or inappropriate.* Practitioners and parents alike often slip into the mode of addressing immediate problems when they really want to be building skills. Leaders of a social skills training group in general, therefore, should try to reduce behaviors that interfere with appropriate social skills use without getting caught up in basic behavior management or discipline. *Focusing too much on correcting or reducing interfering behaviors detracts from the chief purpose of the group and ends up singling out the one or two children who engage in the most problematic behaviors.* If such distractions become a concern, it can be useful to supplement the group therapy with brief individual counseling for the child along with parent involvement to bring the problem behavior under control during group therapy—rather than having to focus both on social skills development and behavior management within the larger group setting.

The example below demonstrates one way to reverse the inclination to focus on inappropriate negative behaviors in a social skills group without interfering with the group process and the goal of building appropriate prosocial skills.

Two of the five group members repeatedly got into arguments with each other and often would yell at the leaders or other group members when upset. The coleaders felt they had to address the yelling and arguing when it happened, but they quickly found that they were devoting so much time to correcting the problem that they could not make it through their planned teaching agendas. They asked a colleague to observe one group session's interactions and make notes on all positive (prosocial) behaviors exhibited by the group members, especially the two who tended to start the arguments. During the next group session, the leaders praised all the members on the skills and behaviors they were doing well on, and they kept a running log on the whiteboard to record instances of the noted positive behaviors during the meeting for the group members (e.g., "Joe waits his turn to speak," "Layla uses appropriate voice volume"). As was the case in this group, the leaders did not need to keep up this approach throughout the life of the group. The participants quickly responded to the fact that positive behaviors were being attended to and the log was not used in subsequent groups. All of the members—but especially the two who were accustomed to being reprimanded and corrected—appreciated the positive attention, and there was no yelling during the group meeting.

During middle childhood and into adolescence, youths who have spectrum disorders often stand out more from their same-age peers because of the things they "don't get." I am referring specifically to the lingo, jargon, sarcasm, and jokes that typically developing adolescents and teens use regularly. Teenagers with ASD usually need to be explicitly taught common phrases that are not meant to be taken literally. It may also be helpful to teach the child some strategies for what to do when he or she doesn't understand what someone is really saying. A boy with Asperger syndrome might, for instance, practice *not saying anything at all* when a peer says something that he is not sure he understands. Or, if it is a close friend and someone he trusts, he might ask, "What do you mean?" In a group setting, it can be helpful to have a whole therapy session dedicated to "understanding lingo." All the group participants could keep a journal for a few weeks before the meeting to record what words or phrases they hear at school that they are unfamiliar with or unsure of the meaning. During the group session, the leaders could help decipher the meanings (using online tools, typically developing peer tutors, etc.) and also teach the participants how to guess at the meaning by using various contextual cues (e.g., the person's tone of voice, what the conversation was about).

A final consideration in focusing on skills development is the importance of making sure that the child understands *why* the specific skill is important. How much explaining of the *why* is needed may vary, depending on the child's motivation and the particular skill taught. For a child who desperately wants to make friends, for instance, explaining that kids tend to want to hang around other kids who are polite and don't interrupt them might be sufficient in trying to teach skills related to waiting for a pause in the conversation before starting to speak. In essence, group leaders should not automatically assume that a child necessarily understands and accepts that a certain skill is important (or worthwhile) and just lacks the ability to use the skill. Sometimes a new appreciation for how a particular skill will benefit him or get his preferences met provides the child with the necessary motivation to learn and master a new skill.

Increase Social Initiations/Responses

This strategy might be considered the heart of most social skills training programs. As such, there are many specific exercises and activities that can be used to help teach initiation/response skills. A list of such activities, along with related handouts and materials, is provided at the end of this chapter.

Some of the general tactics, or considerations, in teaching appropriate social initiation and response skills include using naturally occurring reinforcers, "shaping" the targeted behaviors through rewards, and providing basic scripts (as needed) for the children to follow. If a group member initiates a conversation with a peer or a group leader, then ideally the other person will respond by following the child's lead and not ignore or immediately try to change the topic right away. This type of interaction exemplifies naturally occurring reinforcement: the child with ASD appropriately initiates a conversation on her topic of interest; in responses he gets to talk about something of interest with the peer tutor (positive reinforcement). As with shaping any targeted behavior, initial attempts might not be particularly refined and in fact can be quite awkward or even offensive. However, in almost every social initiation a child undertakes, there is something he did right. If nothing else, at least he tried to initiate an interaction with another person! Group leaders should be mindful of this accomplishment and give specific feedback on what the child did well or appropriately. Consider the following example of both following the child's lead and shaping the targeted behavior:

[The group is having a snack and enjoying free time. Most of the group members are talking about a new video game that was recently released.]

MARTA: That game rocks! My cousin has it, and I played it when I was there last weekend.

SAM: I haven't played it, but my parents said that I might get it for my birthday. I hope so.

MARTA: Yeah—I think my mom will buy it for me.

TONY: [who has been observing but not interacting with peers] My birthday is in April, and I want a new bike!

MARTA: Mine is in April too.

HUONG: Not me—not 'til after Christmas.

In this example, Tony initiates into the group, but his contribution is somewhat awkward (in a loud voice and made abruptly), and what he says is not directly on the topic of the other kids' conversation. However, Marta and then Huong respond—not really about what he says, but on the topic of birthdays. The group leaders should then reinforce and praise Tony's attempt to join the group and comment on what they saw that they liked. They should also provide Tony with tips on how to improve the skill. Sometimes, asking the peers—in this case, Marta and Huong—what they thought about how Tony initiated can be helpful, too. Following are further examples of how the group leaders might usefully follow up on this conversation to make it a true learning experience for Tony:

Example of praising Tony for trying to initiate

"Tony, I like that you tried to join Marta's and Sam's conversation. I noticed you didn't interrupt them—you waited for a natural pause to join in."

Example of giving corrective feedback to improve the skill

"I think that what could make it even better is if you tried to make sure that what you say is related to what the other kids are already talking about a little more. What else might you have said to join into their conversation that would have been a bit more on topic?"

Example of asking the peers to give specific feedback

"Marta and Sam, what did you notice about how Tony approached you or what he said? How did it feel to you?"

Finally, basic scripts that can be followed to practice social initiation can be helpful. Scripts have a long history in the treatment of people with ASD (see Krantz & McClannahan, 1993). Scripts are often taught in the context of individual therapy or counseling but can also be quite successfully learned and practiced within a group setting. For a child who rarely speaks up in a group or initiates with his peers, the leader might provide a script consisting of "Hi—how was your day?" to use at the beginning of the session as the other children enter the room. A verbal script—in which the group leader instructs the child on what to say, and then models it—might be sufficient, or the child might need to have a written script. If so, the leader will want to work on gradually fading the script (i.e., removing specifically required words from the script over time) regularly and on monitoring whether the child continues to rely on the script for initiating or uses more spontaneous unscripted initiations. Children can be taught the basic phrases for greetings, for example, or for talking to a new peer. For detailed information on developing, using, and fading scripts, the McClannahan and Krantz (2005) volume is an excellent source.

As with starting and maintaining conversations, ending them in socially appropriate ways is usually also a focus of interventions with youths on the autism spectrum. Youths with ASD will abruptly end an interaction with someone or just seem to "fade out" of the conversation when they are unsure of how to continue talking or no longer want to talk about a particular topic. After providing some explanation of *why* appropriately ending a conversation is important (e.g., so that you don't appear rude or bored with the person) and ensuring that the child agrees to some degree that this skill is relevant to him or her, discussing some appropriate versus inappropriate ways of leaving a conversation can be helpful.

Again, as with many of the approaches discussed, I tend to either write these out on paper or ask the child to do it so that we have a visual reference. Identify appropriate and less appropriate ways to end a conversation with someone. Then model an *inappropriate* way to end a conversation with the child. See if he or she can verbalize how it felt—odd, rude, disconcerting, etc. Then give the child an opportunity to end the conversation in an appropriate way. Here are some socially appropriate ways to end conversations that might be practiced:

- [If in person] Tell the other person you need to go do something else, and then say good-bye.
  - *Example*: "I really have to get to class now. Nice talking to you."
- [If on the phone] Say something to let the other person know you wish to end the conversation *before* hanging up.
  - *Example*: "I guess I'd better get going. I will talk to you later." [Pause; wait for the other person to say good-bye or something else.] "Bye." [Hang up *after* the other person says good-bye.]
- [If not sure whether the other person wants to end the conversation] Ask the person, offering him or her a way out.
  - *Example*: "Do you have time to talk? Do you have to get going?"

Reduce Interfering Behaviors

Inappropriate behaviors need to be addressed to the extent that they interfere with developing and using appropriate social skills. Key approaches to accomplish this aim include making the group's rules clear at the very start, using differential reinforcement (e.g., commenting when the child demonstrates good listening skills while ignoring minor disruptions), and making sure that group leaders are consistent in their responses to appropriate and inappropriate behaviors.

Whenever I organize a new therapy group, I dedicate time during the very first meeting to review in detail "group rules." Children and teenagers expect this type of emphasis since they are used to it at school. For many therapists, however, this approach may seem quite odd—imposing rules on clients is not something they typically do!. However, considering that we are dealing with a group format and with children on the autism spectrum, providing this type of structure so that clients know what to expect and how to act can have a very positive impact. Not only does it provide the children with clear expectations and information on what the group is all about, but also it can provide a sense of safety and cohesion. This latter benefit is most pronounced when the rules relating to privacy, confidentiality, and mutual respect are clarified.

Another approach that can prove helpful is to develop a group self-monitoring system. An example of one such system my colleagues and I have devised is depicted in Figure 4.1. I explain to the group members that they will be in charge of monitoring their own behavior during each session. They assign ratings to themselves based on how well they interacted during the session, participated with their peers, and followed group rules. In the first group meeting, I let the children, as a group,

FRIENDS' GROUP

Session:	1	2	3	4	5	6	7	8	9	10	11	12
Max	☺	●	☺									
Arnold	☺	☺	◆									
Bradley	◆	●	◆									
Leo	☺	—	⇧									
Andre	⇧	⇧	☺									

☺ = nearly perfect, followed rules, good participation   ⇧ = I should try harder next time

● = pretty good, but I can improve next time   ◆ = rough day, didn't do my best

FIGURE 4.1. Example of a group self-monitoring system.

vote on how they want to do this (e.g., whether to use letter grades, a color code system, or other symbols). Most of the kids really enjoy this self-rating ritual, and the resulting chart serves as a very useful visual reminder of their progress from week to week. In fact, keeping the monitoring chart prominently on the wall for easy reference during each session doubtless spurs better performance from the participants. Very often the children and their parents talk about the "grades" they got that day after the session, and this commentary serves as a good launching pad for a more detailed discussion of what happened specifically during the session. Some parents also use their children's self-ratings as "points" toward selected rewards following the group session, like going to a restaurant that evening or awarding the child free time.

In addition to having clearly established group rules and self-monitoring grading mechanisms, I think it is also important to try to understand what motivates the typical behavioral concerns that group members express or exhibit. Think of this tool as a modified functional assessment (see Chapter 2). Use of this tool is most effective in groups with two coleaders. After the first couple of meetings, the coleaders might meet to discuss the selected skill development targets as well as any behaviors that might interfere with socialization for each child. Sharing observations and discussing hypotheses about what factors seem to be contributing to and maintaining the problem behavior guides the intervention and how the group content is delivered. For example, one child might act up for attention, whereas another child might act inappropriately in order to be excused from the group (i.e., motivated by escape). An example of a brief, relatively unstructured individual assessment based on observational data from the first two group sessions is provided in Figure 4.2 (a blank version is in the Appendix, Form 4).

Promote Skills Generalization

One of the main limitations of social skills training interventions for youths with ASD, including group-based programs, is poor generalization. In other words, a child might learn the targeted social skills and apply them appropriately in the therapeutic setting (e.g., in group sessions) but not apply them successfully at school or in other social settings. The following suggestions should promote the generalization of skills, but they do not guarantee it. The generalization of treatment effects is difficult, and it is also of utmost importance. Without explicitly focusing on ways to promote generalization, the actual impact of any social skills intervention may be minimal. Here are some considerations to keep in mind:

Child: Jackson _____ Age: 8 years, 2 months _____

Social skills concerns/goals of parent/caregiver: No friends, teased because he is so distractible and stands too close to others

Social skills concerns/goals of child: Teasing by other kids at school

Observations of the child during group sessions (e.g., likes, dislikes, interests, strengths, deficits): Likes praise and acknowledgment, easily distracted by environmental stimuli, especially likes talking with other group members during free time/snack period

SOCIAL SKILL TARGETS:

Skill/behavior	Teaching strategy to be used	Strategies for at-home practice	Rewards/other considerations
Initiating with peers	Teach specific introduction scripts	Practice scripts with parents and sister	Free time (10 minutes) for every practice session, one per evening
Maintain appropriate personal space	Education about personal space needs, role plays	Observe people at the mall and at school—how close/far do they stand apart when talking?	Praise for maintaining appropriate space

BEHAVIORS THAT INTERFERE WITH APPROPRIATE SOCIALIZATION:

Behavior/concern	Antecedents (precedes, prompts behavior)	Consequences (follows, reinforces behavior)	Possible intervention/teaching strategies
Gets out of seat, walks around room, looks out of window	When something seems interesting, catches his eye	He gets called back to his seat, gets attention from other kids and group leaders	Teach self-monitoring strategies, reminders before group or class to stay seated, points may be earned for staying in seat appropriately

FIGURE 4.2. Example of a functional assessment for a child following two group sessions.

- Including typically developing peers in the group is normally help-ful. Peers model age-appropriate language and behavior, and they tend to give direct feedback—including their immediate reactions to the behavior of others (e.g., "You interrupted me just now—that's irritating!").
- Using multiple "trainers" is generally beneficial and involves having more than one "leader" teach skills or prompt the child, including peer tutors in the group, or integrating parents and others (e.g., siblings) into skills teaching and practice. The child should not become dependent on any one person to provide a certain cue or script stimulus.
- If a skill is taught and practiced during the group session, ideally that skill should be practiced outside of the group (through home-work assignments) and with other people in the child's life, such as a parent, sibling, or another child in the community.

In promoting generalization of skills and maintenance of treatment gains after the group ends, a final consideration is how the termination of the group is structured. A social skills group with similar peers can be a very powerful experience for many youths with ASD. They have met similar peers and often, for the first time, felt accepted and safe around people their own age. It can be hard emotionally for the kids to say good-bye to one another and to their group leaders at the end of the therapy. It also represents a wonderful learning opportunity in that children need to learn how to manage difficult emotions involving peers and friends and how they can take steps to maintain friendships outside of adult-structured activities.

It can be helpful to start talking about how many weeks are left of the therapy in advance of the last session. It also is generally a good idea to set some ground rules for appropriate ways to maintain contact with friends made during the therapy after the group ends. Sometimes children with ASD inadvertently "force" their friendship on others, such as when they request a peer's phone number rather than offering their own first. Or they seem to not understand that they might accidentally hurt someone's feelings, for example, by asking for just one peer's phone number in the presence of all the other group members. The group lead-ers might broach the subject of the group's termination a couple weeks in advance by saying something similar to the following:

> "After tonight, we have only two more meetings together. That means that Thursday after next is our last group session. I am sure going to miss seeing all of you each week.

Next week we will plan a special party for that final meeting and spend some time talking about what we have learned. We will also talk about what to do if you want to stay in contact with any of the other kids in this group. It is okay with us if you hang out outside of the group if your parents are okay with that. But there are two rules. First, please don't ask for anyone's phone number or email address. If you want to talk to someone, give that person your number or email address instead. Second, if you do offer someone your contact information, make sure you do it when it's just you and the other person present so that you don't accidentally hurt someone else's feelings. We will talk more about this matter next week."

Finally, during the last group meeting I like to have a special "closure" activity—ideally, something that will help the children consolidate the skills they have learned in the therapy and also allow them to create something tangible to take with them as a reminder of their experience in the group. One option is creating memory books to summarize the skills covered during the therapy. This exercise can be a fun activity for the kids and is quite simple to plan. Using materials such as colored pencils, markers, construction paper, and staplers, each child gets to create his or her own "book" made out of several sheets of folded paper stapled at the side. The leaders instruct the children on how to title each page:

- My name is ...
- One of my favorite things to do is ...
- Some of the kids I met in this group are ...
- One social skill I tried to improve is ...
- One thing I think I really improved ...
- One skill I will continue to work on ...
- Two ways I will keep working on this skill are ...
- Anything else I want to make sure I remember from the group ...

Considerations When Constructing a Group

Build Comfort and Rapport in the Group

Before starting a therapy group, the group leaders should determine the focus of the group (i.e., overall goals for teaching, or content) and discuss the desired group dynamic (process factors). Although skills groups are conducted with a clear purpose in mind—to develop the members' social skills—and tend to have much more structure and didactic teaching than open-ended process groups, they are still *therapy* groups. Group therapy can be rewarding—but also complex and challenging, at times. Leaders need to have a shared understanding of the individual group members' needs and histories and make the effort to develop a sense of group cohesion and support within the social skills group.

One simple way to promote such a sense of cohesion and openness is through the use of limited self-disclosure from the leaders about social difficulties they have experienced. A leader sharing with the group, for example, how she often felt "left out" when she was in high school because she wasn't terribly popular models an appropriate level of personal sharing and can encourage the other group participants to disclose their own social difficulties. Of course, leaders have to be careful about how much they share and make sure that what they do disclose is relevant to the other group members. Peer tutors can also be quite powerful "models" of self-disclosure. A major benefit of the group format is having one's peers available for mutual support and learning. Without being able to feel safe and comfortable within the group, this major benefit is lost.

Level of Functioning

If there is just one key statement that is true for all individuals on the autism spectrum, it may be this: *There is enormous variability in functioning among individuals who have ASD.* Clinicians who organize groups must consider factors beyond diagnostic subtype when selecting group members. Ones facility with the spoken language, how much language the person understands, and overall maturity level (in addition to chronological age) should be considered. In addition, group leaders should consider the amount of inappropriate, maladaptive behavior that can be tolerated in the group. For example, will children who have tantrums or manifest severe aggression be acceptable as group members, or should they be enlisted in a different group or type of therapy? Trying to limit the heterogeneity of the group membership in certain respects can aid learning and cohesion.

Girls versus Boys

The gender composition of the group is often a consideration. Since there are many more males than females diagnosed with ASD (approximately a 4:1 ratio), it can be challenging if not impossible in some clinical contexts to develop groups to address the needs of girls with ASD specifically (i.e., a girl-only group). There is some evidence that being the sole girl with ASD in a group-based intervention with boys can be an adverse, even isolating, experience (Barnhill, Cook, Tebbenkamp, & Myles, 2002). Among older children and teenagers, the interests of boys and girls can sometimes diverge radically. It can also be a concern when a member of the group struggles with sexually inappropriate behaviors (e.g., pulling pants down). However, I have conducted many groups composed of both boys and girls, all without much difficulty. It can, in fact, be useful to have same-sex and opposite-sex peers to practice skills with, since kids interact with both boys and girls in other settings such as at school. In sum, mixed-gender social skills groups can be highly useful and are often necessary (e.g., owing to the difficulty in developing a group with only girls), but group leaders should always be mindful of the circumstances that might inhibit the success of such a group.

Who Are the Group Leaders?

There should be at least two adults in the room to serve as coleaders, for three main reasons. First, multiple instructors can help in improving the generalizability of learned skills, as noted earlier. Second, having two leaders is often useful for logistical reasons—if one leader suddenly needs to step out of the room with a child or set up a game or activity, teaching activity can continue uninterrupted with group members. Third, the social interactions between the leaders can serve as useful modeling. Leaders are constant models of appropriate social interaction: their social behaviors with each other and with group members are exemplars of how to behave. In order to demonstrate appropriate male–female interactions—a skill that so many young people with ASD seem to have difficulty with—it may be preferable to have one male leader and one female leader. But this arrangement is often not possible, and, based on purely anecdotal experience, I believe that the gender of the leader(s) does not have much overall affect on the children's level of participation or outcomes. Both group leaders should have some knowledge of ASD, experience in interacting with people with ASD, and previous exposure to group therapy.

Troubleshooting Problems That Arise during Group Sessions

No matter how many preventive or antecedent-based approaches you adopt, there will still be times when problems with interfering behaviors arise. The severity of the behavior and especially how disruptive it is to the group generally determine how (and whether) to address it within the group session. In one session that I conducted, one boy repeatedly put his hand down his pants. This behavior, clearly inappropriate, upset the other children, distracting them from focusing on the session's lesson. My coleader and I discussed the behavior afterward (i.e., its antecedents and consequences; see Figure 4.2) and subsequently asked the child's parent about it. Our conclusion was that the boy was not purposely trying to be gross or disruptive but rather that he lacked an understanding of appropriate and inappropriate places to engage in the behavior. He did not understand or appreciate the distinction between public versus private behaviors. This particular behavior also seemed to be a habit for him, something he did when bored or not really engaged in what was happening. However, the behavior was quite disruptive to the group— the other children got distracted or sometimes laughed or yelled at him, telling him to stop. To address the problem we developed a nonverbal signal (i.e., placing hands on lap) to cue the child when he looked like he was about to engage in the behavior. The signal was discreet and didn't interrupt the flow of group interactions. Of course, we praised him for decreasing the frequency of the behavior, and he was proud of that accomplishment. Although this particular behavior was successfully addressed in the group, it is worth noting that the child continued to struggle with engaging in "private" behaviors while in public locations. His mother found that creating individualized "Social Stories" (discussed at length in Chapter 5) related to specific behaviors that were concerning proved quite helpful for him.

In another example, a girl in a social skills group repeatedly used obscene language during group sessions—mainly when she was excited or wasn't sure how to interact with her peers. For this behavior, a three-strike rule worked pretty well. The first offense in any given session would just draw a warning. If the offense were repeated, she had to step out of the room for 1 minute. If she swore a third time, she was sent out of the room for the remainder of the session. This strategy worked well with her because she was highly motivated to be in the group with her "friends." In fact, she never "struck out" and had to be removed from the group for a whole meeting. This consequence-based strategy was also combined with teaching her "replacement" behaviors, or skills that helped her interact with her peers more appropriately. Since it was clear, from our observational assessments, that she was most likely to swear when excited or confused, we taught her first how to recognize when she was starting to feel this way (self-monitoring) as part of an emotion recognition/monitoring instruction module taught to the whole group. Her identified replacement behaviors included relaxation strategies (taking two deep breaths) and voluntarily taking a brief break from the group interaction to collect her thoughts (she would ask to use the bathroom).

Strategies for Improving
Appropriate Social Initiating and Responding

There are a number of activities or games group leaders can use to help group participants practice initiating and responding to interactions in common social situations.

Checker Stack

This activity can be carried out using any board game pieces, poker chips, or other tokens. The object of the game is to practice conversational turn-taking and the skill of "staying on topic" during a conversation. One child starts a conversation on a topic of his or her choosing and lays down a checker. The peer then responds and puts a second checker on top. Typically, the other children in the group can serve as the audience, and if either person's comment is off-topic or not in turn (e.g., monologue speech), that person does not get to lay a checker down, and the game then starts over.

My colleague (K. Koenig) and I have also developed this activity into a competition of sorts in which the group breaks into various "teams" of two players each, with the members seeing who can accumulate the highest checker stack. In this version of the game, each child gets at least two turns with different conversational partners. One option is to allow the player or team with the highest checker stack to choose that day's snack or free-time game.

Starters and Connectors

Children in the group can be taught very short phrases or scripts for starting a new conversation (e.g., "Hi—what's up?") and "connectors" for keeping the conversation going. Connectors are usually nonverbal signals, like nodding your head, or a one-word comment ("Neat") that shows you are interested. Both starters and connectors are practiced in the group so that each person gets to practice both. It can be helpful to have several starters and connectors written on the whiteboard for the first practice round and then fade them out. See how things go when the visual reminders are taken down or erased. Some children need reminders, such as one leader giving a subtle verbal prompt of what they might do or say.

This activity can be used in a group format or in individual social skills training. I especially like when someone (either the conversation partner or therapist when this exercise is done in a one-on-one format, or another member of the group) can keep track of when the person uses connectors. A peer in the group, for instance, might jot down a hash-mark on the whiteboard or raise one finger to signal whatever one of the connectors is used.

- *Example starters:*
  - Wave at a person subtly; nod your head if he or she is nearby; smile; say "Hello" or use another greeting.
- *Example connectors:*
  - Nod your head; smile; raise your eyebrows slightly; lean forward; ask a simple question (e.g., "Was it fun?"); use a one-word comment (e.g., "Neat").

Joining a Group

After reading brief stories about children joining a peer social group, using skills incorrectly and then correctly, teach and practice the following two steps: (1) look for a cue, and (2) say something! We teach some common nonverbal cues to watch for that indicate it is okay to join (e.g., someone smiles at you, someone looks at you or waves you over to talk) and cues that say "Don't join," such as when two people are whispering to each other or arguing, or you aren't familiar with what they are talking about. The group members add cues to both sides of the list—"Join" and "Don't join" (see below). If the cues indicate it is appropriate to join, the second step is to say something to initiate into the group. Several age-appropriate and very brief phrases or greetings are reviewed (e.g., "Hi, I love that _____ [movie, etc., what peers are talking about]").

Cues that say "Don't join."	Cues that say "Join."
• People are whispering.	• People are smiling.
• You don't know what they are talking about—or anything about the topic they are discussing.	• You are familiar with the topic of conversation.
• People are arguing.	• Someone in the group looks at you or smiles at you.
• Others that members add.	• Others that members add.

Conversation Ball

This is a fun game that combines conversational skills and physical activity. Each person gets a turn to start a new conversation on whatever topic he or she chooses to so long as it's age-appropriate and potentially of interest to the other people in the group. The person who starts the conversation then asks a question or invites someone else in the group to join the conversation and then throws the ball to that person. Each person then follows the same rules, in turn. The object of this activity is to practice conversational turn-taking, contingent conversation, and joining into conversations as well as picking up nonverbal conversational skills (i.e., using visual cues). The ball provides a visual reference for where the conversation is flowing. The game requires everyone to pay attention, even when not talking, because you don't know when you will be thrown the ball next. This game can be played for as long as is helpful during the group session, but every person should get at least one turn to start a conversation. If one child seems to be excluded from the conversation, the leader can subtly enter into the conversation (e.g., put hands up to request the ball and make a comment) and then pass the ball on to the child who had not been included.

Modifications to Conversation Ball can include (1) keeping it totally silent (to focus on nonverbal cues only, such as modulated eye contact); (2) requiring that each person say the name of the person whom they are addressing (helping group members to learn one another's names); and (3) creating a competitive aspect by requiring that if a player makes an off-topic comment or hesitates too long when holding the ball, he or she has to sit down until the next round.

What to Say to Peers

This activity is designed to help group members identify ways to start conversations with new or unfamiliar peers. We first identify three to four "safe topics" and then practice some of the basic skills to use when starting conversations. This type of activity is good for children who don't necessarily need to follow scripts but who struggle with knowing what to say to someone or who tend to start conversations on topics that are not always appropriate. I have found it especially helpful for kids who have a tendency to launch into highly specified or personal topics with peers. The first step is to help group members identify some broad topical areas that are probably good for most social encounters with peers. Some possible safe topics include:

- A recent or upcoming event from school or class (e.g., the test the children just took, next Friday's football game)
- Weekend plans (e.g., if a peer has any fun things planned)
- Favorite sports, teams, or games
- One's activities during a holiday that just passed—or last weekend, if it is a Monday

The identified topics are written on the whiteboard for the participants to refer to during practice. Before the practice component of the group begins, the group leaders discuss some of the basic conversation initiation skills—the "signs" to keep in mind:

- *Signs to look for*: Pay attention to the other person's signs, or indicators, that they are open to talking to you. These are things like eye contact, a smile, or looking around the room.
- *Signs to show others*: Smile, make eye contact, or use other nonverbal greetings (e.g., a head nod) to initiate interactions.

Each group member identifies at least one situation they are likely to encounter in which they would like to be able to start a conversation with a peer. These situations are then practiced, in turn, with the other group members taking on appropriate roles.

CHAPTER 5

Strategies for the Classroom

Perhaps the strongest argument in favor of including students with a disability such as autism in the regular education curriculum and classroom is that the mainstream social milieu enhances social development in children with ASD (Dahle, 2003). However, if children with ASD do not receive sufficient guidance and opportunities for social success with normally functioning peers, the potential benefits of being with non-ASD peers are often not realized (Mulick & Butter, 2002). The strategies outlined in this chapter are all intended to promote skills development with typically developing peers in the traditional public school setting, and these strategies can be implemented within the regular educational curriculum.

Most students with ASD who are considered "higher functioning" are not in full-time special education classrooms. These students are usually in the general education curriculum or sometimes in "partial inclusion"—in which most or part of their day is spent in the regular school classroom. If the student is identified by the school as having autism, she may have an IEP, which outlines special services and accommodations granted to help her succeed academically. Accommodations often seen in students' education plans include extra time for tests and assignments, preferential seating, and provision for special therapies (e.g., speech therapy, occupational therapy) for a certain amount of time each week. However, it is unfortunately uncommon to see an IEP for a higher-functioning ASD student that includes measurable objectives related to social competence or that has specific strategies in place for promoting improved socialization skills. These shortcomings, however, are not necessarily the fault of the educational system or the student's teachers and counselors.

Simply put, schools have thus far not been given a lot of help in this area. Most teachers, counselors, and school administrators truly *want* to help these students do well—not just academically, but socially as well. But the reality is that there are very few intervention approaches that are known to be efficacious. *Given that the typical school day is already filled to capacity with academic demands in a high-stakes environment that emphasizes accountability, carving out time specifically for social skills training is extremely difficult.*

In light of these competing forces—the need for efficacious strategies that teach social skills to students with ASD at school versus intense competition for teachers' limited time and resources—it is imperative that school officials and teachers become more knowledgeable about approaches to social skills training that can be readily incorporated into the student's general education curriculum without undue strain on either time and resources. Either the school counselor, the student's appointed advocate or aide, or the regular education teacher can implement strategies. This chapter covers three related topics: considerations in assessing social skills deficits in students with ASD in school; general approaches to interventions in the school setting; and specific strategies that can be incorporated into the classroom.

Assessing and Understanding the Problem

Before addressing specific strategies, it is important to fully understand the typical social problems of a student with ASD, including what is causing social difficulties, factors that may be maintaining or contributing to the difficulties, and what has previously been tried to improve the situation. These are the basic requirements of a functional assessment (Hanley et al., 2003), a systematic procedure for determining the cause(s) of an identified behavioral concern. The general approach for conducting a functional assessment was provided in Chapter 2. Briefly, functional assessment is based on applied behavior analysis, which assumes that *all behavior is purposeful*. It is conducted in order to identify what contributes to or precipitates the target behavior (antecedents) and what follows the behavior and therefore might be reinforcing it (consequences). Based on this information, hypotheses are formed about the behavior (e.g., the student seems to be making inappropriate sounds to get peers' attention).

In a school setting, the school psychologist normally conducts this type of assessment and then shares his or her hypotheses with the student's IEP team. In an educational setting, sharing one's understanding of the dynamics underlying the behavior is extremely important because many people are involved in the child's education and any prospective intervention—his or her teacher(s), parents, or the school counselor, for example. Many children and adolescents with ASD can benefit from actively participating in the assessment of their problems. Students with ASD may be taught how to help in conducting a fairly unstructured assessment of the antecedents and consequences of their targeted problems. Figure 5.1 shows a sample filled-in template for the student's use (a blank version is included in the Appendix, Form 5), on which the child records his or her observations about the targeted skill or problem as

WHAT is the problem? I get lost during a lecture and don't know how to ask questions—or if I should ask questions. Then I get more upset and want to leave.

WHEN is it most likely to occur?	History class, algebra class
WHERE is it most likely to occur?	School
In what SITUATIONS is it most likely to occur?	Before tests, when new material is being taught
BEFORE it happens .. (antecedents)	I started getting nervous that I won't understand the material. I think about I shouldn't even be in these classes—they are too hard.
AFTER it happens ... (consequences)	I get more nervous, sometimes I start sweating and the other students notice. Sometimes I ask to leave to go to the bathroom, then I get more lost when I come back to class.

Possible hypotheses to explain this problem or behavior: Worry and anxiety about not keeping up in class is distracting and actually contributes to getting more lost in the material, because I can't focus on what the teacher is saying.

What is one thing I might do to improve the social skill or behavior? Try to calm down at the start of class and focus on what the teacher is saying. Don't ask to leave!

FIGURE 5.1. Modified functional assessment for student's use.

well as hypotheses and ideas for strategies to improve the skill. Normally the school psychologist or other person responsible for the intervention will help the student complete the form the first couple of times. Then, as new behaviors are targeted, more responsibility is given to the student for completing his or her own functional assessment. *The aim underlying this type of student involvement is twofold, namely, to get the students' input on the problem or issue unfiltered, or directly, and to give them practice in thinking about their problems in a highly functional and problem-solving way.*

Following the assessment, such interventions as modifying either the antecedents or the consequences and teaching the child a more appropriate skill to get the same need or goal met are put into place, and then further observations are made. This cycle is repeated until the behavior is under control or at least is much improved. In addition to helping to solve problem behaviors, functional assessments can be usefully employed in better understanding social problems and in teaching social skills.

The tenet that all behavior is purposeful is just as true for misbehavior as for appropriate conduct. Once the behavior of interest is understood through the functional assessment, the goal is to decrease any behavior that impedes appropriate socialization or integration with peers (e.g., nose-picking) and replace such actions with more socially acceptable conduct. Theoretically, teaching actions that result in the same desired outcome (e.g., attention from peers) should result in adopting the new behavior in place of the undesired behavior *if* the new behavior successfully results in the desired outcome as quickly as the old, unacceptable behavior and does not lead to unwanted consequences.

Intervention Approaches

Visually Based Strategies

Visually based teaching strategies offer many advantages in successfully teaching social skills to students with ASD. Many children on the autism spectrum relate much more readily to visual learning methods than to auditory ones (McCoy & Hermansen, 2007). For these youngsters, visual cues and reminders can be quite salient and useful. In addition, many strategies can be implemented relatively unobtrusively in the classroom without being obvious to other students, and they can be used repeatedly. A child with ASD can refer back to the visual cue or story, for instance, as frequently as he or she needs to before performing the skill.

Video modeling, a visually based intervention that has received empirical support for increasing children's socially appropriate behaviors (Nikopoulos & Keenan, 2007), can be successfully adapted for use in a school setting for such matters as adjusting oneself to a new classroom (McCoy & Hermansen, 2007). This strategy can also be used in clinical settings and by parents at home, making it very helpful for promoting generalization in that the same approach can be used to teach a skill across multiple contexts. Video modeling is especially appealing to many youngsters with ASD because of their natural attraction to high-tech gadgets. Watching a scene on television or on the computer screen is inherently more appealing for a lot of kids with ASD than watching it enacted live or reading about it. The fact that the modeled lesson or scenario can be viewed over and over again is also an advantage since many children with ASD appreciate repetition and need multiple teaching trials. There are many situations in which it is desirable to demonstrate expected and appropriate behaviors before the child is actually prepared to confront the real situation (e.g., a school dance). Modeling can be very helpful for students with fluency deficits (see Chapter 1) in that they may largely have the knowledge but yet struggle with successful implementation. The video often depicts the skill in action; and occasionally it can be helpful to demonstrate the skill being done both incorrectly and then the correct way.

Ideally, the actors or models in the video should be similar to the target student in age and other characteristics. Depending on the student and the specific targeted skill, the actor/model might be a peer, a sibling, or even the student himself acting out the targeted skill (McCoy & Hermansen, 2007). The videos need not be lengthy, at most about a minute long. Also, teachers and parents could work collaboratively to create videos for the students' needs. The teacher might create the first couple of videos, and then parents could help to create more videos, as needed. Video modeling has been combined with such other intervention techniques such as *in vivo* skills training (Haring, Breen, Weiner, Kennedy, & Bednersh, 1995) and reinforcement (LeBlanc et al., 2003) to further improve outcomes.

As an example of video modeling, a child might feel anxious about the start of the school year or about going to a new teacher's classroom. The parent and teacher together could create a short video in which the teacher of the new classroom greets students in her classroom and the students respond appropriately, to demonstrate what the class will look like and what the students are expected to do. The student could watch this video repeatedly at home during the week before school and then practice it live with the teacher before the first day of school—that is, before other students are present.

"Social Stories," developed by Carol Gray (1998, 2000), is another visually based strategy. Unlike so many treatment approaches that target skills acquisition and the learning of appropriate social behaviors, the goal of Social Stories is to develop the child's *understanding* of social relationships and events—the who, what, when and why of our social world. Once created, the stories can serve as reminders of what to do in a given situation. The stories are brief narratives describing specific social situations; they are individualized for the child and written from the child's perspective to make the instructive content meaningful to him or her. The primary purpose of Social Stories is to teach and explain a concept or situation, rather than discrete social skills. Possibilities for the content of Social Stories are endless. For example, a story might be written for a child about deciding which entrée to select at lunchtime and then informing the cafeteria worker—or even one about waiting to be called on by the teacher.

Stories can be quite simple—some consist of just two to three sentences—and can include illustrations as simple as stick figures with attached, hand-written labels or captions. They can also be more formalized and elaborate. Sansosti and Powell-Smith (2008) developed an intervention that used both Social Stories (in PowerPoint) and video models, presented via computer. In the described intervention, the children first read the Social Story and then saw the targeted skill or behavior being enacted by the model. In general, when introducing a new story to a child, the teacher (or counselor, or the like) might simply say, "I've written a story for you. Let's read it together." Other people the child likes—perhaps a parent or older sibling—can reread the story with the child to promote consistency. It is preferable to also have some Social Stories that are not about skills deficit areas. Starting with stories about the child's strengths or prosocial behaviors provides an opportunity to praise him for a behavior he already demonstrates, and it can make working on the more difficult skills a little easier. Gray (2000) has written a highly user-friendly book with many sample Social Stories that can serve as a valuable resource. Two sample Social Stories are included in Figure 5.2.

Self-Management Techniques

Approaches in this domain can be applied across such diverse settings as the classroom, the home, or the wider community. Children can often be taught to monitor their own behavior in relation to a particular goal. For example, following small-group or individualized training in *social initiations*, the teacher might initiate a self-monitoring plan with the student. There are many self-management techniques available—including use of a wrist counter or paper-and-pencil checklist—that the student can use to track the frequency of the targeted behavior. A younger student

Sharing

I may try to share with people. Sometimes they will share with me.

Usually, sharing is a good idea.

Sometimes if I share with someone, they may be my friend.

Sharing with others makes them feel welcome.

Sharing with others may make me feel good.

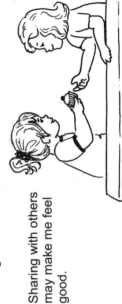

Receiving a Treat in School

Sometimes someone will give me a treat at school.

It might be something to eat for a special occasion. We may have treats to share the fun of a classmate's birthday. We may have treats to celebrate a holiday.

The person who brought the treat has to make sure that there are enough treats for everyone.

When someone gives me a treat, I will try to remember to say, "Thank you."

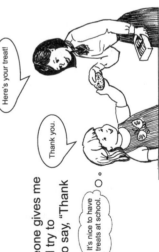

FIGURE 5.2. Sample Social Stories. From Gray (2000). Reprinted with permission from Future Horizons, Inc.

might keep the tracking checklist taped to her desk; a student in middle school might keep it inside a folder he carries with him to classes. Some students may find it too arduous a task to carry the checklist with them and remember to track their behavior throughout the day. When this is so, one should designate blocks of time during the day when they can do the tracking—such as at the end of the lunch period and/or on the bus ride home after school.

If the goal is increasing the frequency of initiations while at school, one simple approach might be to keep track of the number of initiations the child makes by recording hash marks in his folder. Each day or week the target is raised gradually (e.g., two initiations, then three initiations), and the teacher provides reinforcement (such as extra free reading time), for appropriate self-monitoring and progress in (or attainment of) the targeted goal. For many students, it is helpful to meet with the teacher at the end of each day to review the monitoring sheets. This brief meeting can be an opportunity to praise the student's effort and send positive notes home to her parents on progress made. Such feedback, if given on a daily basis, can also keep the student motivated. As a supplement to the self-management system, parent-delivered reinforcement can be built in. If both the student and the teacher agree that the student met his goal (e.g., five appropriate social initiations with peers on a given day), for instance, the parent might choose to reward the child with a special treat that evening, such as a dessert of his choosing.

Parents and teachers sometimes express concern about using rewards (e.g., the dessert) in this context because of a fear that the reward will be the sole motivation for the socially appropriate behavior—that the child is not intrinsically motivated to improve social skills but rather only demonstrating the skill so as to reap the reward. This concern is understandable; however, use of external rewards can be quite helpful in spurring change. In addition, based on my own experience, most of the higher-functioning children with ASD with whom I have worked desire to improve their social competence. *It is not motivation, but rather skill, that they lack.*

For those students who are not terribly motivated to be social and improve their own competence in this domain, research has demonstrated that a structured reward schedule can be useful. Koegel, Koegel, Hurley, and Frea (1992) used a self-management approach to increase social initiations in school-age children and found that, even with rapid thinning of the reinforcement (i.e., the reward given after several appropriate initiations), sustained improvements in social initiations were recorded. Moreover, they found that pairing tangible reinforcers such as edible treats with social reinforcers (e.g., attention, praise) actually increases the salience of the social reinforcer. Eventually the tangible reward can be faded out so that only the social reward is given. Indeed, the appeal of self-management techniques is that they help transfer responsibility to the child and yet are self-sustaining. Some extra work and external reinforcement may be needed at the beginning, however, to make them effective if the student is not initially self-motivated to master the skill. An example of a self-monitoring record sheet involving tangible rewards is shown in Figure 5.3.

Skill: _____

Mark in each box [✓] every time you use this skill. At the end of each day, you get to choose your reward!

> 2 checks = I get to stay up 15 minutes later at bedtime!
> 3 checks = I get to choose dessert!
> 4 checks = Game of my choice with Mom or Dad!
> 5 checks = Special outing on the weekend with Mom or Dad!

Monday:

Tuesday:

Wednesday:

Thursday:

Friday:

FIGURE 5.3. Example of a self-monitoring recording sheet.

Peer-Based Strategies

Most structured social skills interventions are directed by adults, although the goal usually is improved interaction with the child's same-age *peers*. As such, over the past decade research in this area has devoted progressively more attention to social behavior in natural settings (e.g., the classroom) and with typically developing peers. Indeed, peers are often full-fledged co-interventionists (see Rogers, 2000 for review)!

There are many advantages to peer-mediated interventions. Skills may be more readily generalized to other situations, contexts, and children than with interventions using only adults as instructors and partners. Incorporating peers into social skills training is highly proactive and, depending on the type of intervention implemented, can result in fewer demands on the teachers' planning time. This approach is easily adaptable to the classroom and generally promotes a positive helping atmosphere in that environment. However, most research studies of peer-mediated approaches have been conducted with preschool-age children. More research is needed to understand the most effective ways to implement peer-based strategies with older students. New research initiatives in this area are especially important, given that so many adolescents with ASD experience greater difficulty in socializing with same-age peers than they do with younger children or adults.

Interventions employing normally functioning peers vary greatly in how they are structured and in the roles that peers play. At the most basic level, the arrangement fosters a classroom atmosphere of friendly collaboration in which students help one another. The teacher can assign students to work jointly on projects, ensuring that each student with ASD is paired with a socially skilled and empathic peer partner on group projects and that no student is excluded by classmates. One must avoid letting the classmates select the "teams" or groups for projects, as that approach might leave a student with ASD as the last person chosen. In other words, when larger working groups are called for, a method other than student selection (e.g., group assignment based on sequential numbers, names drawn out of a hat, or teacher assignment) works best.

Other relatively informal pairings or groupings involving peers include lunch groups, usually designated by the teacher or another adult, and classwide buddy systems. Laushey and Heflin (2000) described a buddy system implemented with kindergartners in which the teacher rotated how students were paired each day. The children would check to see with whom they were paired at the start of each day for such activities as free play or recess. If such a system were implemented classwide, all the students would be instructed on how to interact with their buddy (e.g., "Stay with and talk to your assigned buddy"). For older students, such pairings might be most feasible in specific classes or sections that were relatively unstructured, like physical education or study hall. Of course, if a student were singled out or expected to help another student with ASD on an ongoing basis, that student would need adequate training on what to do and what to expect from the student, and the teacher would need to secure his assent as well as his parents' consent to such longer-term peer mentoring.

Peer involvement can enhance socialization in students with ASD even when the focus of the intervention is *not* on social skills. Kamps, Barbetta, Leonard, and Delquadri (1994), for example, found that social interaction increased during free time and academic performance increased immediately following peer tutoring/instruction in which typically developing students were paired with students on the spectrum.

Peers might be taught how to model certain skills, how to initiate with a child with ASD, or how to prompt appropriate behavior from the child. Using peers in intervention and training necessitates considering the degree of confidentiality within the environment (e.g., after-school group or the school classroom itself), and the parents' desires with regard to sharing information about their child. Depending on the nature of the intervention and the preferences of the student with ASD and his parents, information on ASD might be provided to the peers.

When first introducing a student with ASD to classmates, care should be taken in choosing the source—that is, specifically who is sharing the information and how the information is conveyed. Morton and Campbell (2008), for example, found that older students (fifth graders) responded more favorably in terms of their subsequent attitudes toward peers with ASD when the information about the autism was provided by a doctor, whereas for younger students (third graders) the child's mother was more readily received. These researchers concluded that it is probably most beneficial for students to receive information about ASD from multiple sources (Morton & Campbell, 2008). Basic information on what the spectrum disorders are as well as awareness of associated strengths and problems may help peers be more understanding of and sensitive to their classmates.

Campbell, Ferguson, Herzinger, Jackson, and Marino (2004) reported that providing both explanatory information (e.g., "Joe's behaviors are due to a biological condition that he can't control") and descriptive information to highlight similarities between the child with ASD and his peers can be effective in improving peers' cognitive and behavioral attitudes toward a student with autism. As with any disability, the decision of how much information to disclose to a student's classmates or even whether to disclose it can be difficult. Concerns about stigma and negative attitudes compel some parents to choose not to tell the other students or sometimes even their child's educators or school officials. On the other hand, disclosure about the disorder and appropriate education about ASD may contribute positively to improved communications with the school authorities and more supportive peer relationships as well (Campbell, 2006). One example of how a teacher might introduce a child who has autism and explain the disorder to the class follows. This example assumes that the family has given their approval and consent to share such information.

> "Class, I would like to introduce Rudy to you. Rudy moved here from Glendale Elementary School. He likes soccer and video games, and he is really good at spelling. Rudy also has autism, a biological disorder that can make it hard for him to get along with his peers sometimes and to make friends. Rudy can't help it, though, and he wants to make friends. If anyone has questions about autism, he or she can ask me. Let's all welcome Rudy to our class."

Other Strategies and Activities That Can Promote Social Integration and Skills Growth

Environmental Changes

Brown, Odom, and Conroy (2001) recommended that socialization interventions be delivered hierarchically, starting with the least intrusive and progressing in terms of intensity based on observations of the child's skills development. One of the least intrusive (and often overlooked) strategies involves environmental modifications intended to promote social integration with peers. Relatively simple adjustments can sometimes facilitate social integration in the classroom and promote the use of appropriate social skills. Teachers can structure the curriculum and the classroom to promote social interactions by situating the student with ASD so that distracting stimuli (e.g., ambient road noise from the open window) that contribute to inappropriate behaviors are minimized, providing lots of opportunities for cooperative learning and mixed social group activities, by pairing the student with a socially skilled student during play and academic work, or by arranging desks into small clusters based on the teacher's knowledge of students likely to work well together.

The teacher can also highlight the strengths of the student with ASD or give him a special role in the classroom. The quiet, awkward student with autism might possess highly advanced mathematical skills, for example. To recognize the student and develop his social self-confidence, the teacher might call on him to answer questions about a difficult math problem (thereby highlighting his special skills) or suggest that he help another student who is struggling with math. A cautionary statement is in order here, however. Publicly recognizing such skills can back-fire, such as when the student is self-conscious or when praise from the teacher draws unwanted peer attention or even jealousy.

The student who sometimes gets emotionally overwhelmed in the classroom environment might be assigned the role of "delivery person." When the teacher needs to communicate with the principal's office or have photocopies picked up, she might ask him to go to the office for her. This errand gives the student a socially acceptable break from the classroom routine. When the teacher recognizes that he is starting to feel overwhelmed (perhaps he starts rocking in his seat or looks confused), she asks him to go to the office with a message. This assignment enables him to save face socially so that he doesn't just storm out of the room, gives him a special responsibility, and potentially provides the oppor-tunity for him to practice some social skills (e.g., talking to unfamiliar adults in the principal's office). Of course, this type of strategy can only be used with students who have demonstrated that they are capable of being safe while unsupervised for brief periods of time at school. The teacher should not allow a student who may run away from school or become destructive when upset, for example, to leave the classroom unsupervised.

Drama

Many adolescents on the spectrum seem to enjoy drama or theater. Although there is not a wealth of empirical research on the efficacy of drama as an intervention approach, many young people with ASD have an affinity for theater and the dramatic arts; they enjoy the experience and do quite well in it. Some plausible reasons may be that kids who enjoy theater and drama may generally be more accepting of uniqueness in peers and open-minded. This attitude can create a refreshingly warm atmosphere among peers.

Another factor may be the focus on language and language arts in theater. Words are the primary medium through which expression occurs. For many adolescents with ASD, especially those with AS, there is a special ability to remember what they read and apply "rules" to what people do. It must also be noted that, in a play or musical, one's interactions with the other characters are entirely scripted and directed. There is no guesswork—unless, of course, the play is improvisational. This dynamic is very different from the day-to-day unscripted demands that normal socialization at home and at school typically exacts. When acting in a play (unlike conversing in a small group), there is an audience that *does not respond and to which the child need not respond.* The rules and expectations are clear, the interactions often lack nonverbal cues that the child must follow or interpret, and there are no unanticipated shifts in the conversation he must track.

Whatever the specific differences, thespian activities often prove a fruitful social outlet for students with ASD. Although not solidly grounded in research findings just yet, the experience may help students find an accepting peer group, provide an opportunity for success in an academic and "social" pursuit, and help build their motivation to undertake other more purely social endeavors with classmates.

Skills Training

Formal social skills training can also be conducted either during the school day or after school hours. The teacher or other school officials, such as the school psychologist, might take the lead in organizing the program. A set curriculum can be implemented or portions of various manuals can be integrated to meet the needs of the students in the program. In most schools, it might not be feasible to include only students with ASD in the program, and including students with other disabilities (e.g., specific learning disabilities) can be helpful. In the Further Reading section there are several structured skills training curricula listed for youths with ASD.

Communications between School Officials and Parents

Asking the student's parents about his or her child's social skills, particularly any specific skill concerns they have, can be very informative. Because these same skill deficits are likely to show up in the classroom, having detailed knowledge about them in advance can help the teacher prepare to handle them and consider options for teaching appropriate prosocial replacement skills. Parents also tend to really appreciate a proactive approach on the part of the educator. It shows concern and can set the stage for an excellent working relationship throughout the school year, as the following case example demonstrates.

"Amanda's" new teacher was aware of her diagnosis of AS; so, before the first day of fifth grade, she set up a meeting with Amanda's parents to discuss her difficulties and strengths. From her parents, she learned that Amanda frequently misinterpreted peers' behaviors, which in the past had often led to her believing that other girls did not like her—that they in fact were talking disparagingly about her. Twice

Amanda had been suspended from school because she reacted aggressively when she thought someone was talking maliciously about her. On the other hand, she also learned that Amanda was very socially motivated and had an intense interest in horses—she read about them, went riding on weekends, and her dream was to buy her own horse once she had saved enough money. With this knowledge, Amanda's teacher set up some class projects for the beginning of the year on the topics of nature and animals. Another girl in class shared Amanda's equestrian interests, and they were paired together to do a report on a topic of their choice, which was horses. To try to proactively prevent the behaviors that had previously led to her suspensions, the teacher met with Amanda for a brief "touch-in" after lunch each day to see how things were going and to determine whether she needed any breaks or help (e.g., talking to the counselor) during the afternoon period. The beginning of the school year went quite well, and Amanda seemed to make a good friend in her class who shared her interests.

Communicating with parents about what is happening in the classroom is also imperative. Regular reports home on the progress, problems, and goals of the student are very much appreciated by parents. The student's parents can be invaluable in providing encouragement, practice opportunities, and reinforcement to their child for work done during the school day.

Case Example

A fourth-grade student with autism, "Reggie" was large for his age but very socially immature. Most of his classmates avoided interacting with him because he was so hard to get along with. On several occasions, his teacher and school psychologist observed him in class and at lunch with his peers, and they conferred with his parents about their concerns—that Reggie was too socially assertive with peers, overpowered others on the playground, and insisted on having others do things his way. Reggie expressed a desire to his parents for more friends, but his difficulty with social interaction prevented him from making and keeping friends. Reggie was rigid and socially inflexible. Once he had made a decision about how to do something, it was nearly impossible to get him to alter it. This attitude led to problems in working with classmates. On group projects he would adamantly insist that others do it the way he said, he talked over others, and he would get angry when peers asserted themselves or their ideas. In gym class, he frequently got into arguments with the teacher and classmates about the rules of games or how teams were chosen. These incidents usually ended with Reggie yelling and cursing, being excused from the class or walking out, and going home early. Needless to say, these incidents also led to further rejection by his peers.

With the help of Reggie's parents, the teacher created a brief Social Story that explained the importance of "compromise" in social situations and group projects. Reggie and his teacher read the story together several times, and Reggie kept the story, which was in a small three-ring binder, with him. At home, his parents helped Reggie practice compromise with his younger sister and gave him feedback and praise as he improved.

For Reggie's first "real-life" practice, his teacher devised a small-group exercise in her class that would require the students to work in pairs to create an art project. She talked to Reggie beforehand about the exercise and explained that she would help him as needed and would also monitor how he was doing. She paired Reggie with a fairly popular and friendly student in the class who was unlikely to get too frustrated with Reggie. Reggie struggled mightily in suppressing his dominating ways; fortunately he was able to let the other student have his say in how to accomplish the project, and they finished it on time. Afterward, the teacher shared with Reggie her observations and suggestions and reinforced his admirable effort(s). She sent a note home to his parents summarizing his accomplishment. Reggie continued to refer to his social story, and eventually added more social stories to his binder. The teacher continued to create opportunities in the class for him to practice his social skills productively with his peers.

CHAPTER 6

Strategies for the Clinic

A variety of approaches can be used to enhance social competence in children with ASD who are seen in clinical settings. Although it is often preferable to conduct social skills training in more natural environments (e.g., at school) so that the child has access to peers for practice, there are situations that make individual therapy in the clinic the most appropriate forum for intervention. Some children are not emotionally ready for a group-based intervention or have secondary problems that prevent them from productively being in a peer treatment group. A child who is extremely anxious or aggressive, for instance, often requires individual therapy, at least initially. Once the child's problems are well under control, continuing social skills treatment in a small group then becomes a viable option. Then, too, social skills training groups for children with ASD are not always readily available. In such circumstances, individual counseling or therapy to improve social skills can be quite helpful.

There are many possible formats for social skills training in individual treatment. Often, a child is in ongoing individual therapy and the therapist incorporates aspects of social skills training into his broader treatment program. Individual therapy does not preclude a child from being in another type of treatment to enhance his social skills. The child can have his regular therapist and also attend group therapy led either by his own therapist or another practitioner. This type of adjunctive treatment really does offer the child the best of both worlds: he gets the continuity and individualization of a supportive therapeutic relationship, and he gets to "try out" his newly acquired skills immediately with his peers.

The approaches covered in this chapter are intended for use by a therapist treating a child with ASD in a one-on-one format. These strategies and techniques should be used flexibly, called upon as needed, and integrated alongside other strategies as guided by the child's treatment plan. For youths with spectrum conditions, improving social skills may be the primary target of intervention, or it may be just one of several treatment goals. It is my hope that these strategies can be integrated with other approaches the therapist chooses to use in an effort to address the unique needs of the individual client. This chapter reviews some of the more general treatment approaches that can effectively be used with clients with ASD and then offers examples of some specific intervention strategies (see Table 6.1).

Before addressing psychosocial intervention strategies, I must briefly mention the need to coordinate treatment with the client's physician or psychiatrist, when applicable. Many if not most youths with ASD are psychiatrically medicated, often with multiple medications and often for secondary concerns such as inattention or aggression. Unintended and adverse side effects, variable treatment responses, and unpredictable dosing schedules (e.g., Martin, Koenig, Anderson, & Scahill, 2003) make the involvement of the therapist or counselor—who typically sees the client much more frequently than does the prescriber—a necessity. It is therefore essential that the social skills interventionist be aware of the client's medication regimen and be mindful of the possibility of adverse side effects. Many medications prescribed to youths with ASD, for instance, cause sedation, which can interfere with their ability to participate in an after-school skills training group or attend to individual therapy.

Treatment Approaches

Behavioral Therapy

Behavioral therapy (BT) places primary importance on overt observable behaviors. Intervention approaches based on BT and applied behavior analysis (ABA) have long been the mainstay of treatment for youths with ASD (Schreibman, 2000). Fundamental social skills teaching techniques such as modeling skills, prompting for desired behaviors, and reinforcing appropriate social behaviors share a common foundation in the principles of operant conditioning. One of the most common behavioral approaches used in the context of individual therapy involves shaping closer and closer approximations to the target behavior while simultaneously withholding reinforcement for inappropriate or competing behaviors. For example, a child may initially be rewarded with tokens redeemable for prizes after the therapy hour just for making eye contact with the therapist. As the child's skills improve, more is required—such as asking a question while making eye contact—to earn the tokens.

TABLE 6.1. Strategies for Developing Social Competence in Individual Therapy

Affective education and emotion regulation

- Work on identifying cues (physiological, physical, cognitive, and environmental) of specific emotions.
- Develop a method for the client to measure the intensity of his or her emotion and convey that information to others.
- Identify appropriate strategies for coping with intense emotions (e.g., a coping "toolbox"; Attwood, 2004).

Cognitive restructuring

- Teach how to identify thoughts by using visual cues, analogies relevant to the client, and examples.
- Address the client's tendency, if present, to be overly literal and/or to make false assumptions.
- Teach and practice the scientific method of thought investigation.

Conflict management

- Address theory-of-mind deficits; provide alternative explanations to the client for the behavior of others when misperceptions exist.
- Teach a systematic problem-solving approach.

Psychoeducation

- Normalize the client's experience.
- Educate about ASD—its strengths as well as its deficits.
- Provide corrective teaching (e.g., misconceptions about the nature of friendship).

Developing the client's strengths

- Foster acceptance of diagnosis, including specific strengths and deficit areas.
- Incorporate the client's special interests into the therapy, perhaps as a reward for therapy accomplishments.
- Promote self-efficacy by ensuring that the client can experience success; teach skills in a stepwise fashion.

Specific skills teaching

- Teach didactically with client's learning style in mind.
- Explain the rationale for specific skills.
- Use self-disclosure as needed.
- Model appropriate skills.
- Incorporate practices and exercises into therapy.
- Provide immediate and detailed feedback.
- Reinforce the use of appropriate skills, or at least the clients best efforts.

General strategies

- Foster parental involvement.
- Never underestimate the importance of therapeutic rapport.
- Use homework to promote skill use and generalization.
- Be clear on the therapy rules (e.g., be on time, do the homework, etc.) and on the expectations for the therapy.

In the same vein, if the therapist suspects that attention seeking is the motivation behind a socially inappropriate behavior, she might decide to intentionally ignore the behavior and then immediately re-engage with the child when the inappropriate behavior stops. Such selective but deliberate ignoring is most effective when it is done in a systematic and even obvious manner. The therapist might, for example, actually turn in her chair and avert her eyes completely while ignoring the client and then immediately turn back around to face the child and smile when the inappropriate behavior stops.

Parent Training and Involvement

Parent training (a subject discussed at greater length in Chapter 7) is usually a component of any clinic-based intervention. Parent training has long been employed as an intervention for many core and associated problems of ASD, such as noncompliance, language development, and social skills training (Johnson et al., 2007). A heightened level of parental involvement in the treatment of youths with ASD is needed for two main reasons. First, individuals with spectrum disorders often lack nonfamilial support systems. At times when most people might seek support from friends rather than parents and family, adolescents with ASD usually do not have a peer social support group and instead must rely on their parents for guidance and support. Second, challenges to using skills capably and poor generalization of treatment gains necessitate parental involvement. In the context of child-focused therapy, parents are often needed to help with at-home exercises between sessions and to provide encouragement and reinforcement for their child as he or she works on learning and using new skills. The therapist should educate the parent about ASD and the client's specific challenges and strengths and should be available throughout the course of intervention to answer questions that the parents may have. The importance of parental involvement in individual therapy with the child or teen cannot be overstated, because the parent typically plays such a vital role in the child's social and academic life.

Cognitive-Behavioral Therapy

Cognitive-behavioral therapy (CBT) focuses on therapist–client collaboration and investigation of the client's thoughts, feelings, and behaviors related to specific problems. It may seem counterintuitive to adopt a CBT approach when treating a high-functioning person with ASD, given characteristic difficulties with skills like metacognition and insight. However, there is evidence that CBT can be applied successfully to treat individuals with autism and related spectrum disorders such as AS. Several clinicians and scientists (e.g., Gaus, 2007; Attwood, 2004) have demonstrated that CBT can be adapted to people on the spectrum, and initial pilot studies are confirming positive outcomes (e.g., Chalfant, Rapee, & Carroll, 2007; Lopata, Thomeer, Volker, & Nida, 2006; White, Koenig, & Scahill, 2010). The investigative method and problem-solving approach most central to CBT can be very appealing to the logical, rule-bound way of thinking that is characteristic of many clients on the spectrum.

CBT may be particularly helpful in developing fundamental social competence. Youths with ASD have deficits not only in their knowledge and use of appropriate social behaviors but also in more fundamental skills such as perspective taking, noticing and accurately interpreting nonverbal social communication, appropriately expressing nonverbal behaviors (e.g., facial expressions), and recognizing emotional states in oneself and others. Owing to the complex nature of ASD-related social deficits, the argument for more intensive treatment than merely basic behavioral social skills instruction is a convincing one.

Specific Intervention Strategies

Psychoeducation

Providing information on the child's specific diagnosis often turns out to be one of the most valuable intervention strategies a clinician can offer his patient. I often think of what one 12-year-old boy with AS said when I asked him what he would like to get out of counseling. After thinking about it for some time, he replied, "I would like to be more like a normal person ... and get rid of my social issues and anxiety issues." This youngster knew about his Asperger diagnosis but didn't really understand what it meant or how common the disorder is. More important, he believed that he was *not normal* because he had AS and that "normal" people didn't have trouble with relationships or struggle with anxiety. In situations like this, providing accurate information can be very helpful and normalizing for the youngster. I explained to this particular child how prevalent ASD—like AS—actually is and how almost all people— including those without ASD—often struggle socially and encounter anxiety daily. It took some convincing and presentation of actual data (in this case, figures from studies on the prevalence of ASD and having him survey family members about their worries and anxieties), but when he finally accepted that his ASD didn't make him "abnormal" it was almost as though a heavy weight was lifted from his shoulders. Of course, it didn't make his problems go away or directly improve his social skills, but it did help normalize his feelings and his struggles. He became more willing to engage with peers, which allowed him to practice the skills he was learning.

When providing information to the young client or the parents, I suggest giving as much or as little as is called for at the time. In the beginning of treatment with a new family, I share my diagnostic impressions with the client and the parents and invite them to ask me any questions they may have—about the diagnosis itself, educational and treatment options, etc. Usually I try to ask the parents separately from the child in case there are concerns they have but don't feel comfortable sharing in front of their child. Such concerns are often related to long-term prognosis, how independent the child may become, and alternative (nontraditional) treatments they might be considering. The goal is to let the parents know that I am always available, in case they want information now or if questions arise later in the treatment. Similarly, with the child, I usually explain the disorder by using age-appropriate terminology and use drawings to depict the things she or he might struggle most with (see Figure 6.1 as an example). I ask both the parents and the child at that time what questions or worries they have and tell them that if they think of any questions later they should feel free to ask them at any time.

Another helpful strategy to use in educating clients about ASD is to talk to them about some of the common descriptors of people with ASD.

COMMUNICATION
- I don't understand others' gestures when they talk.
- I sometimes pick the wrong words to say what I mean.

SPECIAL INTERESTS
- I know a lot about racing.
- I have a huge collection of miniature race cars.

SOCIAL DIFFICULTIES
- I want more friends.
- I get picked on at school, but I'm usually not sure why.
- Sometimes the other kids don't want to talk about what I want to do (racing),and I get upset.

FIGURE 6.1. Visual depiction of common ASD-associated concerns.

Form 6 in the Appendix lists some terms that might apply to a person with ASD. I like to present this list to the client during the first session when we discuss spectrum disorders and ask him to circle which terms best describe him and cross out terms that he feels don't describe him. Going through the client's responses to the list of descriptors can serve to model seeing positive and negative attributes in people, including one's self. This is often useful as many clients on the spectrum engage in "all or nothing" thinking (i.e., viewing someone as "cool" or "geeky" with little appreciation for shades of gray in between). It also helps me to get to know the client and understand his self-perception better. Finally, it is a useful tool to exemplify just how different people who have an ASD diagnosis can be, and that there are associated strengths as well as deficits. Psychoeducation is normally an ongoing activity throughout the treatment, and I often find it helpful to answer the client's specific questions about ASD and his or her specific diagnosis as they occur. Direct teaching on related topics is frequently called for, as well. Children with ASD often have an unusual or a mistaken understanding of what friendship really is (Attwood, 2000). For example, some children with ASD might well consider to be their friend a peer at school who picks on them and taunts them but who occasionally talks to them during gym class. Such "friendships" are not the real thing, a fact not always obvious to someone with ASD. Therefore, education on what makes someone a true friend and guidelines for recognizing true friendship can be beneficial to the client.

Providing the Rationale for Skills Instruction

In addition to teaching the basics and implicit aspects of particular skills, such as standing an appropriate distance from others whenever waiting in a line, it is often necessary to teach the child with ASD "why" the skill is important. One should not automatically assume that the child or teen knows the rationale, and just lacks the technical know-how for performing a particular skill. *Many people with ASD need and appreciate explicit instruction and explanation as to why the targeted skill should be important to them.* As a hypothetical example, a teenage boy with Asperger syndrome who tends to talk too loudly in the cafeteria during lunchtime might learn skills related to volume control, such as the difference between an "indoor voice" and an "outdoor voice." Yet, he usually fails to use his indoor voice whenever he gets excited. After his therapist explains why it's important to modulate how loudly he speaks—so that other people can be heard, to show respect to the meal servers in the cafeteria, to avoid unnecessary noise, and so forth—he seems to "get it," and he starts using an appropriate voice volume more consistently.

One approach included in many social skills training programs that can be applied in a one-on-one setting with a child or in a group environment is the use of social vignettes. Different from Social Stories (see Chapter 5), such vignettes are less structured and are usually written in the third person. Vignettes are brief stories about social situations and problems that are used to explain a concept or skill such as social problem solving or conflict resolution. They can then be used as a launching pad for further discussion of social difficulties relevant to the specific child (Bauminger, 2007).

Social vignettes can be used to exemplify both *why* the targeted skill is important and *how* using it properly may help the child achieve her goals. Vignettes are especially useful when working with a client who is defensive about her skills and social difficulties or when the client has difficulty in recognizing the effects of her behaviors on others. Consider the following sample vignette that could be used with a client who desires more friends but exhibits behaviors that turn her peers off and effectively work against her goal of gaining more friends.

"Sarah" was really smart and pretty and did well in school, but she was lonely and didn't understand why the other girls in her school seemed to reject her. She wasn't invited to birthday parties or over to people's houses. Eventually she got so frustrated that she started making up mean jokes about some of the more popular girls. Some of the kids seemed to think the jokes were funny, and they sometimes laughed with Sarah. But in class most of the girls refused to talk to her, and some of them even started moving their desks away so that they didn't have to sit by her."

After reading the vignette together, or telling it to the client, the therapist could follow up with such questions as "Why did Sarah tell jokes about the girls?," "Why do you think the girls moved their desks away?," and "What else might Sarah do to meet her goal of having more friends at school?"

In Figure 6.2, an example of a worksheet that can be used at the start of individual therapy is provided (a blank version is included in the Appendix, Form 7). This worksheet is intended to help the client identify his social strengths and problems, create a shared understanding between the therapist and client as to how some of the problems might get in the way of his reaching his goals, and identify some specific goals to work toward. The worksheet can be used as a tool for the therapist and client to reference throughout therapy in relation to specific social skills. For example, if the child identifies that one of his goals is to have

Everyone has things that they are quite good at or really enjoy doing—and other things that they don't like so much or struggle with. Below we will take some time to write down some of these things.

 Things I am really good at (SOCIAL STRENGTHS):

Video games, games of strategy, singing

Things I struggle with (SOCIAL NEEDS/DEFICITS):

Saying rude things when I don't mean to, understanding jokes

Social difficulties get in the way of . . .	When I have learned and practiced some *new social skills*, I will be able to . . .
Talking to kids at school and making friends	*Call people on the phone, get invited out to do stuff, not be so bored all summer*

Two social goals I have:
1. *Have a friend to hang out with after school*
2. *Hang out with friends over the summer, so I don't get so bored*

FIGURE 6.2. Example of a completed goals worksheet.

someone to hang out with after school, then working on specific skills that progressively help the child both reach this goal and remind him whenever he is straying off course can be highly motivating.

Mind Reading and Empathy

Deficits in the ability to recognize and interpret the thoughts, emotions, and intentions of others (Baron-Cohen, 1995) can have serious consequences for social interaction. Consider the following example. A young girl with PDD-NOS, "Tonya," is seated at the end of a row of desks in her mathematics class. The teacher hands out homework, and the students are expected to take one sheet and pass the rest back to the students in their row. The girl in front of Tonya does not pass the homework back. Tonya becomes furious and yells at the girl, "Why aren't you giving me the homework? You jerk!" Tonya does not recognize that the girl got the last sheet, so there were no more sheets to hand back—that the teacher was one page short for her row. In other words, she misinterpreted an accidental oversight on the teacher's part as an intentional slight from her classmate.

Theory-of-mind skills, or the ability to consider the thoughts and feelings of others, can be improved in people with ASD. Howlin, Baron-Cohen, and Hadwin (1999) developed an approach that teaches skills in a hierarchical fashion by using photographs, pictures, and text to portray emotions. Children first practice identifying people's basic emotions (e.g., from pictures of faces) and then predict the responses and feelings of others based on the depicted situations. The therapist portrays a wide variety of emotions that the children must then interpret until their skills improve.

In therapy it can sometimes be helpful for the counselor to share personal feelings and reactions when they are relevant to the client and his or her developing theory of mind skills. One school-age client I treated, "Arnold," insisted on bringing whatever book he was currently reading into the therapy sessions. He was an avid reader and had an especially intense interest in science fiction books. Before each session, he would read his book while waiting in the lobby and was compelled to finish the section or chapter that he was reading before putting the book down, even after the session started. This practice interfered with his treatment because sessions often started late since I had to wait for him to finish. During one session, Arnold and I were discussing his relationship with his older brother. He was quite upset and felt that his brother was "rude" because he changed the television channel the night before while Arnold was watching a show. I empathized with him and gently tried to help him consider his brother's point of view. Arnold conceded that he had been watching the television for over an hour and that his brother's favorite show was starting. This exchange led to a discussion on how we can sometimes think other people are rude or inconsiderate even when they aren't trying to be. Because I thought it was a relevant teaching example, I gently expressed my frustration with Arnold's insistence on reading even after our sessions started and explained how it made me feel (e.g., frustrated, ignored) even though I knew he was not trying to offend me intentionally. Arnold was surprised at how his habit of reading at the start of our session time adversely affected my feelings and how the same behavior in other situations, such as in class or when visiting a relative's house, also made other people feel peeved or ignored. Arnold and I continued to work on skills related to interpreting other people's feelings and thoughts, as well as on recognizing how a person's thoughts could be affected by what he did or said.

Emotion Education and Regulation

Cognitively higher-functioning youths with spectrum disorders typically have difficulty in achieving real depth in their affective information processing. That is to say, empirical research indicates that many people with ASD, while normally able to recognize and accurately label basic emotions (e.g., sadness), nonetheless struggle with more complex emotions (e.g., embarrassment). As described by Bauminger (2002), this relative lack of knowledge about complex emotions involves aspects of social cognition that people with ASD do not readily perceive. Understanding cultural norms and social rules, recognizing how one should interact with others, and the ability to take responsibility for one's own behavior in a social context (e.g., the experience of guilt or pride) are all involved in affective understanding and recognition. In therapy, the client will often struggle with understanding his or her emotional responses and properly linking one's emotions to various social situations. Several specific issues are frequently encountered in therapy in this domain with the client, including the possibility that he or she might:

- Associate a thought with a particular behavior without recognizing the intervening emotional state
  - *Example*: When asked *how he felt* after an argument with a peer, the client might explain, "I felt like he was being a jerk, so I told him so!"
- Struggle with recognizing and appropriately labeling different degrees of an emotion
  - *Example*: The client might rate his anger as a "10" on a 1–10 scale whenever he is even mildly upset.

- Fail to understand how to interpret internal states and feelings
  - *Example*: The client struggles to label or describe his feelings of sadness; his description appears to be of anger, instead.
- Feel suddenly overwhelmed by the intensity of her negative or positive emotions
  - *Example*: While discussing an argument with her mother during a therapy session, the client suddenly exclaims that she is leaving and walks out of the room, only to return several minutes later offering apologies.

Affective education often occurs alongside cognitive restructuring in therapy. Depending on the nature of the problem, there are many ways to promote affective understanding and improved emotion regulation skills. Many young people need help with first recognizing what the emotion is and then managing the *intensity* of their emotions. Tony Attwood (2004) has written extensively on clinical tools for emotion regulation in higher-functioning people with ASD. One such strategy involves the creation of "books" about specific emotions (Attwood, 2000). A child's book on happiness, for example, might include photographs of the child doing things that make him happy, pictures clipped from magazines of people who look happy, and even reminders of events, things, or activities that make the child feel happy (e.g., a picture of his dog). In therapy, these "emotion books," which are used to identify the characteristic facial features that indicate particular emotions, help the child understand the nature of emotion as occurring along a continuum—that happiness can be small (e.g., when one is pleased) or intense (e.g., ecstatic). The therapist and child typically also identify other emotional "indicators" such as tone of voice, body language, and cues in the environment or the situation. One fun way to practice affect recognition is to make it into a game in which the therapist provides clues (indicators) of different emotions and the child's role is to accurately identify the feeling (Attwood, 2004).

Identifying strategies for emotion modulation and recognizing the contexts in which certain emotions (e.g., extreme excitement) are appropriate or inappropriate are also often significant therapeutic goals. The therapist can help the client develop descriptive words for various degrees of emotion in order to appropriately express what they are feeling (see the case example at the end of the chapter). Broadening the client's affective responses along with their vocabulary for describing their emotions and improving their ability to relate their emotions to their social interactions is often a key clinical objective. The specific coping tools that are chosen should be based on the client's interests and aptitudes. Various options include exercise, relaxation, or spending time engaged in a preferred activity (Attwood, 2004). In my own experience, many children with ASD tend to rely on one tool nearly exclusively and/or dismiss other viable coping tools without trying them. In such a situation, a problem-solving approach (discussed in the Problem Solving section, page 115), in which all the possible strategies (i.e., tools) are identified and considered before evaluation occurs, can be especially helpful. One useful technique is to enumerate the various coping tools on index cards and have the client sort the cards by type (e.g., tools to use at home and at school, tools—like taking walks—that require extended periods of time, and tools that other friends have used).

Improving Flexibility

Everyone prefers to have things their way, including people who have ASD. Youths with autism and related conditions, however, encounter significant problems when they insist on having things "their way" and their rigidity increases. Such impulses likely reflect a need for control and are generally most manifested when peers don't follow their rules in games or assignments or when there is a need for compromise.

This problem can be successfully addressed through individual counseling. First, the clinician inquires whether the client ever has problems getting along with other kids because they don't follow the rules, etc. The aim here is to help the child recognize that his or her rigidity may be getting in the way of attaining significant personal social goals (an approach that both provides a good rationale for employing skill and building motivation). Sometimes children with ASD view "flexibility" as a negative attribute; so, explaining that flexibility often has positive consequences is very important. Flexibility—the ability to "roll with the punches" and accept that unexpected things sometimes happen—is an important life skill. It helps us function better with other people in school and in life, and it helps to avoid getting too stressed, which is unhealthy. At this point, it is useful to ask the child about his or her thoughts on flexibility: "What does it mean to be flexible? What is hard about accepting and then dealing with change? What happens to you when things don't go as you planned?"

The clinician then demonstrates flexibility by using materials familiar to the child. This tack can be taken via a Social Story, self-disclosure of personal experience, or such other means as a video clip, book, or television show with which the youth is familiar, that shows characters behaving in flexible and appropriate ways. Discuss with the child how flexibility (e.g., compromise, turn-taking) was used in the example and how this situation turned out. Finally, specific skills for improving flexibility are taught. One approach to do this is to use *skill cards* with the child—several index cards that describe specific skills. One skill is listed on each card along with a brief example of how or when the skill might be used. Listed below are examples of specific flexibility skills. Which skills are taught depend on the individual child, what skills he or she already possesses, and what situations are most problematic for the child.

- *Self-talk*: telling yourself something internally as a "reminder" to help you cope with the unexpected (e.g., "I hadn't expected this, but I can do it").
- *Relaxation techniques*: breathing, focusing on something else (i.e., a deliberate distraction), guided imagery.
- *Taking turns*: when other people want to do (or talk about) something different from what you want to do (or talk about). Offer to first do their thing and then try yours.
- *Compromise*: meeting in the middle.
- *Wild card*: ask the child to come up with his or her own strategy. It might be an adaptation on one of the skills already covered or it might be something completely different. Possibilities include taking a break from the activity to "regroup" mentally and then rejoining the activity or conversation—or developing a "mental image" of flexibility (it might even be a cartoon character!) as a reminder of how to act.

After several skills are identified, the clinician should model how to put one or more of the skills into practice. Then the child in turn practices by first describing a situation in which he or she could use the flexibility skill and then role playing the situation with the clinician. Ideally, the child would be able to identify times or situations in which the need to be more flexible could be practiced *in vivo* (i.e., real-time in the real-world setting).

I like to give the cards to the child to take home to practice with. It can be helpful for him to jot down, on the backs of the specific skill cards, notes about when he used the skill and how it went. Flexibility training can be implemented in a group therapy setting as well, and this exercise can be especially instructive when the child is able to practice interacting flexibly with peers. Role play can be used best to re-enact the particular situations that are most problematic for the child. One young lady I worked with, for instance, would get really upset and angry when her classmates did not listen to the teacher or follow classroom rules. She would "tell" on her classmates to the teacher—or even reprimand them as though she were the teacher. This pattern of behavior, of course, generated a lot of negative flack from peers. In the therapy group she was able to use her peers to practice acceptance and tolerance for other students' behaviors. Skill cards, as used above, can also be integrated into a game format. For example, if five or more "flexibility skills" were identified in the group, the members of the group could take turns drawing from the deck of skill cards and acting them out, similar to charades, for the other group members to guess at. The only limitation is the therapist's or group leader's imagination!

Cognitive Restructuring

Helping young clients understand how their thoughts affect both how they feel and how they act is a core focus of CBT. Recognition of unhelpful and distorted thoughts (e.g., "This is absolutely awful!"), developing more helpful and adaptive thoughts about the situation (e.g., "I wish it were better, but it's not the end of the world"), and recognizing one's emotions are all typically addressed in interventions based on CBT. Sze and Wood (2007) outlined several adaptations to traditional CBT for children with ASD, including reducing the use of abstract language and placing more emphasis on strategies such as role playing and visual teaching materials, incorporation of the child's special interests into teaching and creating examples, and a highly interactive (as contrasted to didactic) teaching style.

In my own experience treating children and adolescents who have ASD, I have found it is typically helpful to first spend some time making sure the child can generally distinguish among thoughts, feelings, and actions and then discussing how the three are related—that changes in one (e.g., a thought) can affect another (e.g., how we feel). Visuals intended to demonstrate these relationships—such as cartoons or drawings on the whiteboard—can be helpful to many children. I try to have the child develop her own definitions of thoughts, feelings, and actions in ways that she can remember and talk about readily with me and with their parents. A simple handout (see Figure 6.3 and Form 8 in the Appendix) can be helpful in this regard.

When explaining distorted, unhelpful types of thoughts, I try to find examples and analogies relevant to the child. One I particularly like is the analogy of a bug in a computer program:

> "Errors in thinking are kind of like bugs in a computer program. If a program has a bug, it doesn't always run right. It might get the wrong answers or overlook certain types of data. Similarly, if I have an error in how I think, it might get in the

Thoughts are things we tell ourselves about things or people. Some examples of thoughts I have:

"I can't do this"

"No one is like me"

Any special way I can remember how to distinguish a thought?

Like a thought bubble cartoon, the words I tell myself that no one else hears

Feelings are emotions that can be felt throughout my body. Some examples of feelings I have:

Nervous, scared, fidgety

Any special way I can remember how to distinguish a feeling?

Comes on suddenly, makes it hard to concentrate

Actions are the things our bodies do when we have thoughts *and* feelings. Some examples of actions I do:

Stomach-ache, sometimes I cry, call my mom to get me, rock back and forth, start

reciting the words to my favorite movies

Any special way I can remember how to distinguish an action?

Actions take energy and are usually noticeable to other people

FIGURE 6.3. Example of a completed worksheet on distinguishing among thoughts, feelings, and actions.

way of the things I want to do or make me ignore certain types of information."

Providing examples like this as well as naming some of the common cognitive distortions (e.g., catastrophizing) can then help the child to recognize his own distorted or unhelpful thoughts. Doing this in the context of a particular situation the child has experienced is usually more effective than trying to have the child think about thinking "in general," which is more abstract (see the next case example). It should be noted that some children with ASD are better able to understand the relationships among various thoughts, feelings, and actions and to think about their own thinking (i.e., metacognition) than are others. For some young clients who can't readily grasp or apply the concepts, even after the counselor uses the relevant examples, visual tools, and so forth, a more behavioral approach in which the cognitive component is not emphasized as much might well be more useful. Over time, these youths may become more capable of fully understanding their thoughts and actions. Some of the more common types of distortion and their brief descriptions are enumerated below. Either prior to or during the therapy session, it may be helpful to list on paper the child's particular cognitive errors as a personal reference guide and make a copy of it for the client to keep for between-session practice.

Common cognitive errors in ASD

- *Jumping to conclusions/catastrophizing*: "I automatically assume the worst without considering all the facts."
- *All-or-nothing thinking*: "Only perfection or a "perfect score" is good enough; anything less means I am a failure."
- *Overgeneralization*: "If something bad happened before, it will happen again."

Restructuring or changing the original thought that occurs to make it more realistic and more helpful to the client is the primary goal of the therapist. Help the child to develop an alternative thought about the situation that might be true, and together consider the evidence for and against each of the thoughts, the unhelpful one and the more helpful/adaptive/realistic thought. What makes the first thought more likely to be accurate? What about the alternative thought? Encourage the child to think like a scientist, considering both sides, what other people might think or do in the situation, and "try on" both thoughts during therapy to see which one feels more "comfortable." Many youths with ASD are quite skilled at logically analyzing a problem in this way. After investigating both thoughts or interpretations thoroughly, I usually ask about how accurate each thought is (in other words, how much the child believes it to be true) and how he would feel if he believed thought 1 versus thought 2.

Figure 6.4 provides an example of a worksheet that can be used in therapy to help the young client investigate her thoughts (a blank version is included in the Appendix, Form 9). When trying to help the youngster identify her distorted thoughts and beliefs and challenge her thinking, modifications often need to be made to accommodate the child's learning style and vocabulary. The examples provided here will likely need to be modified to fit the individual client. The goal, however, is always to help her to recognize when her thoughts are counter productive to achieving her social and other goals and to develop healthier and more helpful ways of thinking about common situations.

Thought to investigate:

"No one will like me at my new school"

How much do you believe this thought or belief to be true and accurate? Rate it below, with *0 being completely untrue* and *100 being absolutely, without a doubt, true and accurate.*

Rating: 90

Now it is time to look at the evidence for and the evidence against this thought. *When doing the investigation, try to answer such questions as: Has this happened in the past? Does this happen to other people? Are there any other explanations?*

Evidence supporting:	Evidence not supporting:
I didn't have any friends at my last school. They will know I am different, that I have Asperger's	The people at my old school knew me when I was younger and hadn't learned better social skills. I have made a couple of friends outside of school, so I know I can do it.

Considering all the evidence *for* and *against* this thought/belief, make another rating of how much you believe the thought to be true and accurate.

New rating: 45

If you lowered your rating at all, try to pick which cognitive distortion is most likely at work:

Jumping to conclusions, overgeneralization

FIGURE 6.4. Examples of a completed investigating thoughts worksheet.

As a therapist, you should model investigative thinking and encourage social experimentation (e.g., an outing into the community to observe others' reactions), as needed. You might say:

"For a child who insists that other kids never talk to you—an example of 'all-or-nothing' thinking—I suggest that we test this belief by sitting out in the lobby together where there are other children, or that we take a walk to the nearby playground and just observe what the other kids do."

Chances are that during such an excursion at least one child will smile at your young client or maybe even say "Hello." Cognitive restructuring is not a single-use strategy; it is often repeated throughout treatment and applied to various specific problems. Gradually, however, the therapist can step back as the child becomes more proficient at recognizing his automatic unhelpful thoughts and developing more realistic and productive ways of thinking about his situation.

Problem Solving

Teaching clients how to solve problems effectively is a key component of many cognitive-behavioral treatments. Instruction in problem-solving techniques can often be effectively applied to social problems and is useful in developing social interaction skills. Situations in which a problem-solving approach might be useful include determining how to handle repeated teasing from a classmate, talking to a new student in class, and finding a place to sit at lunch in the crowded school cafeteria. Although many approaches are available for teaching problem solving, most involve a particular sequence of steps that the problem solver should take (Kendall & Suveg, 2006).

Usually the child is taught to, first, recognize the problem, be specific about defining it fully, and decide what the goal should be in solving it. Problem solving teaches the child to slow down and think through his or her options rather than reacting impulsively (e.g., with a temper tantrum or by avoiding interaction). Possible strategies to address the problem are identified and evaluated. Then a strategy is chosen and implemented. The final step involves evaluating how things went—that is, was the problem solved?

In individual therapy I have found that teaching the steps of problem solving and then applying the approach to a particular problem the child is experiencing is the most useful approach. The child and I talk about the situation in detail and practice each step during the session (e.g., through modeling and role play), including a discussion of how the situation turned out. The child is then usually assigned to use the problem-solving skills in the actual situation outside of therapy. Afterward, usually at the start of the next session, we talk about how things went, if the child's goal was met, and what might need to be adjusted to make things go better next time. An example of using a problem-solving worksheet to help manage teasing at school is given in Figure 6.5 (a blank version of the worksheet is included in the Appendix, Form 10).

1. What is the **problem?**

I get picked on during recess at school. Two boys in particular, Allen and Mike, call me mean names and they sometimes push me. I usually end up crying and running back inside the school.

2. What is your **goal**?

I want the other kids to not pick on me.

I want to not cry in public.

3. What are your **reactions** (physical sensations, feelings)?

I feel hot and I start to cry, my stomach starts to hurt like I'm going to get sick.

Worried, embarrassed

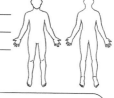

4. What **thoughts** are you having?

They are going to do something and everyone will laugh at me.

I want to leave. I want to go home.

This is awful. They will never stop!

5. A more **helpful thought** for solving this problem: I wish they wouldn't call me names or tease me, but I know it's not just me that they tease. I've seen them bully other kids too. Most of the other kids on the playground don't even notice what is happening.

6. Develop a **strategy**: I will go to a different part of the playground and make sure I am close to one of the adult monitors.

7. **Evaluate**: How did you do? Time to reward your hard work!! I walked away from Allen and Mike when they started being mean. I noticed that it felt like I might cry or be sick, so I walked to a different group of kids. I felt better—I did it!

FIGURE 6.5. Example of a problem-solving worksheet (applied to teasing at school).

Increasing Self-Efficacy

A social learning paradigm is often applied to social skills interventions (Bandura, 1994). In terms of social skills development, this paradigm holds that the child's beliefs about his interpersonal abilities will affect how he interacts with others. If a child thinks he is popular and socially skilled, for example, he is more likely to initiate interactions with new peers and speak up in class than if he believes he is socially incompetent or disliked by peers. Modeling, encouragement, stress management, and reinforcement are mainstays of social learning approaches (Bandura, 1994). The therapist's own self-disclosure can be a social learning experience for the child. By talking about how he or she resolved a dispute with a coworker, the therapist can normalize feelings of frustration and model appropriate problem solving.

In teaching social skills to a child with ASD, the therapist should always be mindful of the extent to which the child typically experiences success. *In their daily social lives, relatively few youths with ASD get the opportunity to be successful.* Teaching skills hierarchically, even starting with simple skills that the child might already be quite adept with, is a good approach to use in therapy to help gradually build self-efficacy. Early on in the intervention it might be useful to set up situations that will guarantee at least *some* degree of success—having the child introduce herself to a colleague of the therapist, for instance. Even with youths with very poor social skills, there are usually positive social behaviors they possess that can be highlighted. That the child came to the session to talk to a stranger in and of itself can be quite hard; commenting on this accomplishment and how impressive it is can go far in building the child's self-efficacy.

Drama-Based Techniques

Drama-based treatment techniques have been implemented with some success to improve the social competence of youths with disorders other than ASD (Glass, Guli, & Semrud-Clikeman, 2000). Although such strategies have not been rigorously tested to determine effectiveness in cases of ASD, anecdotally such approaches have merit. Many specific activities fall under this category, and the therapist can easily integrate such techniques into a more comprehensive treatment approach. In addition to helping to build awareness of nonverbal communication and improved emotional expression, such techniques can be used to move beyond an impasse in therapy and to hasten engagement.

Mirroring is one example of a drama-based technique. The client and the therapist (or another child) practice mirroring each other's facial expressions or body movements silently as a way of practicing recognition of body language and attending to the nonverbal aspects of communication. Clients can also be given "roles" to act out, perhaps in conjunction with the use of socially relevant stories. The child is given a specific role in the story to portray. If the therapist has access to audiovisual equipment, recording skits or role plays and watching them in a later session can both be fun for the client and enhance his or her learning. Another way that I like to help the child develop an improved understanding of how nonverbal behaviors affect social communications is to watch selected scenes from age-appropriate movies or videos *without the sound.* Instruct the child just to attend to what the characters do with their bodies and faces, and see whether they can guess what is happening in the scene while the sound is muted. More often than not, the client is surprised by how much information is conveyed by people's hands, eyes, faces, and bodily movements. Afterward, a discussion of the various nonverbal communications that have been observed is highly useful, and this strategy can also easily be used as a practice exercise at home.

Activity-Based Techniques

Structured activities and games can facilitate social engagement in therapy. By using the naturally occurring interests of the young client with ASD, such as drawing, building, or a particular board game the child enjoys, the therapist can enter into the child's world in a sense. Moreover, engaging in a preferred activity of the client's is usually enjoyable for him or her, thus making it more likely that the client will participate in other collaborative activities and feel more at ease during therapy.

One activity-based technique that has been studied for improving social skills in high-functioning youths with ASD is Lego therapy (LeGoff, 2004). In Lego therapy, the client and others (e.g., peers, the therapist) work together to construct a Lego project. There is a clear division of tasks, such as engineer and builder. To successfully create the final product, the pair or group must communicate, collaborate, and problem-solve together. Preliminary research on Lego therapy as a social skills intervention is promising in terms of improving social deficits specific to autism (e.g., avoidance of eye contact, resisting physical contact) and decreasing maladaptive behaviors (LeGoff, 2004; Owens, Granader, Humphrey, & Baron-Cohen, 2008).

In sum, preferred activities (e.g., trading cards, an interest in construction or architecture) can be used in therapy in creative ways. Perhaps the most obvious way is as a reward for effort during the therapy session. The therapist allots a few minutes at the end of each session, for instance, for the child to engage in the preferred activity. This free period of time can be helpful in ensuring that the session ends on a positive note and in bringing the client back to a "baseline" emotional state, particularly if difficult skills or emotionally challenging material has been covered during the session. Integrating the preferred activities or games into the therapy session can have many benefits, including greater engagement by the client, enhanced rapport, and an opportunity to practice the target social skills in the context of entertaining and fun interactions.

Consider the following ways to integrate preferred activities and interests of the child into the session:

- Use brief segments of time devoted to preferred activities or discussion of the child's favorite topic(s) as rewards following difficult exercises or activities.
- For children who have particular difficulty in staying engaged during a full session, consider breaking up the therapy hour by building in time (e.g., 10 minutes) for a preferred activity or personal interest midway through the session. Include this free time in each session's agenda, as it can work well in signifying the "halfway" point.
- Teach by using examples that involve the child's interests and metaphors that the child can readily relate to (e.g., computers, car racing, animals, etc.)
- When the child is "stuck" in trying to learn a certain skill or reluctant to practice it, consider developing a special reward (even outside of the session, one that the parent can deliver) involving the interests of the child. For example, each time the child practices the new skill at home, she gets extra time with her favorite game.
- When teaching via modeling or social vignette, incorporate the child's special interests into the content of the story whenever possible.

Social Stories, Comic Strips, and Scripts

Social Stories (Gray, 1998), discussed in some detail in Chapter 5, can be incorporated into individual counseling to promote learning appropriate social skills and understanding social situations. One of the main advantages of this approach for use in individual therapy is that the stories can be easily adapted to fit the changing individual needs of the client. By first observing the client in several social situations that are problematic, the therapist identifies specific skills that should be taught through the stories. The therapist can also interview the child's teachers and parents to both understand which social deficits are most problematic. The therapist might create a Social Story that uses the names of peers the child has identified in a very specific situation for the client. Parents can learn the approach and continue to work on Social Stories for their children outside of therapy (Dodd, Hupp, Jewell, & Krohn, 2008). A Social Story often includes text and pictures (which can be drawn by hand by the therapist). Multiple stories can be developed to address several very specific situations or deficit areas (e.g., Sansosti & Powell-Smith, 2006). When several stories have been created, they can be assembled into a book, flip chart, or folder. A three-ring binder works well for portability so that the child can refer to the stories outside of therapy. Resources supplying more information on how to create Social Stories are provided at the end of this volume in the Further Reading section.

Comic strip conversations, also developed by Gray (1994, 1996), offer a useful way of visually demonstrating the various levels of communication that can occur simultaneously. Briefly, using colors to depict emotions (e.g., pink = happy, blue = sad), the child and therapist develop a comic strip that includes thought and speech bubbles. The colors chosen for the text can represent the emotion behind the words (e.g., **"I wish my mom wouldn't say that about my dad"** [written in bold black letters, indicating feelings of anger]). Examples from Gray's (1994) book of how the therapist might draw conversational elements, such as listening or speaking in a quiet voice, in a comic strip conversation are included in Figure 6.6.

A related teaching approach involves the use of predetermined social scripts. Similar to the lines one might get to read in a play, a script provides the words to use in a given situation. There is considerable variability in how this strategy can be implemented. The script can be highly structured, providing the child with exactly what he should say, or just a series of "prompts" to cue him. Scripts are audiotaped or printed words, phrases, or sentences and can be presented as written cue cards, a sequence of words in a binder format, or a page with the script to follow for more advanced learners.

For children with ASD, scripts can be a simple, quick, and relatively inexpensive way to teach skills such as social initiation, conversational speech and turn-taking, appropriate things to say, and strategies for staying on the topic of a conversation. After a script is learned and practiced, the script is gradually faded, that is, the words of the script are erased or removed over time so that the child becomes less prompt-dependent. Theoretically, scripts may be an effective teaching method because of behavioral chaining, in which one response (e.g., the first word of the script) cues another response (the next word), ultimately leading to the end or the reinforcer (e.g., the response from the conversational partner)

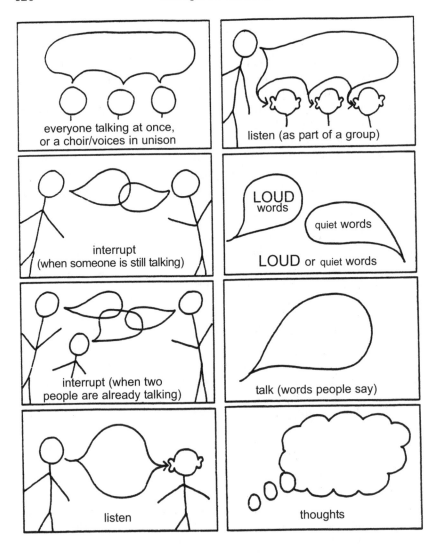

FIGURE 6.6. Guidelines for comic strip conversations. From Gray (1994). Reprinted with permission from Future Horizons, Inc.

(McClannahan & Krantz, 2005). The ultimate goal in teaching is for the child to develop spontaneous unscripted speech. As McClannahan and Krantz (2005) observe, after learning with scripts children will normally continue to use similar scripts that are no longer physically present, combine scripts to make new statements, or use independent speech that they did not learn in a script.

Clinical Considerations

In addition to the content of treatment, including the specific treatment approaches used, there are several more general clinical considerations in treating youths with ASD. Anticipating some of the potential problems and pitfalls and attempting to address them at the beginning of treatment is always preferable to addressing them only after the problems arise. The first goal in therapy should be orienting the patient to therapy and familiarizing him with your respective roles in the relationship. The therapist should anticipate that the child might have some degree of difficulty with the therapeutic relationship, especially if the child is entering her very first therapy experience. A child with autism may not know what to expect, how to act, or even why she is seeing you. In general, a matter-of-fact approach in which the therapist gives simple, honest explanations is helpful. The following is one example:

> "Your mom wanted you to come in today to talk with me because she is concerned about some problems you've been having with other kids at school lately. I am a counselor, and I work with kids when they are having problems like yours to try to find better ways to get along with other kids—so that school isn't so frustrating."

Depending on how the child responds—if he has questions, seems confused, or wants more information, you should provide more details on the nature of the therapeutic relationship and why he is seeing you. Providing information on the rules of the therapy and the expectations for both the therapist and client can be especially helpful.

A second major concern expressed almost uniformly by clinicians who work with persons with ASD is poor generalization of treatment gains. This concern is what I refer to as "the frustration of the 50-minute hour." A child might appear to learn a new skill quickly (e.g., greeting others politely) in therapy and even demonstrate the new skill to her parents at the end of the session. However, the following week, you observe her in the lobby before the session. Although she is seated between two other same-age children, she does not greet them or even acknowledge them nonverbally. Instead she sits quietly reading, with no indication that she is even aware there are other people present. When you ask the parents what has been happening in the intervening days since the last session, they report that she has made no attempt to greet others and, in fact, acted quite inappropriately when a new peer tried to befriend her in dance class. There is no easy solution to this problem, unfortunately. *It is generally accepted that the best outcomes occur when intervention is intensive, takes place across multiple settings, and involves multiple trainers.* As such, therapy that occurs once a week in a clinic may be insufficient to produce lasting change or skill improvement across contexts (home, school, etc.) in multiple skill domains. This is an important point and should be emphasized: *It is generally accepted that individual therapy can be quite helpful but probably is insufficient to address all of the child's presenting concerns and produce positive meaningful change across contexts that will endure without supplementary intervention and other types of therapies.*

To improve the chances that real clinically meaningful gains will be made and maintained over time, there are several things the individual therapist can do. Assigning practice (homework) for the child to do between sessions is important. The child simply *must practice* what is being taught during the individual sessions in the "real world". Ideally, this practice would occur through adjunctive group training, school-based supports, and/or practice on a regular basis that is prompted or reinforced by the child's caregivers. The therapist should also intentionally incorporate generalization sessions into the treatment program. For instance, some sessions might be conducted in the child's community or school following the more didactic skills-teaching component at the therapist's office or clinic. Teaching skills related to dining etiquette might be followed by a dinner out with the therapist in a public restaurant. Of course, such an excursion must be undertaken with the knowledge and consent of the child's parents and be fully explained to the child ahead of time. Another option may be to conduct certain training at various alternative sites. For example, sessions might be held in the therapist's office instead of the clinic, the child's school (after school lets out, when no other students are present), and in the child's home (especially if social difficulties at home are identified as a target of treatment).

Involving other people in the treatment can be difficult—especially for clinicians in private practice—but nonetheless it is quite beneficial. Similar to approaches that involve exposure for anxiety concerns, practice with other people might directly follow teaching sessions. After teaching the child how to incorporate nonverbal communication skills (e.g., smiles, gestures) with language ("hello") when introducing himself, the therapist and child might visit the offices of colleagues in the same office suite to practice the new skill. If the new skill involves interactions with strangers or other children, the child might spend a period of time in the lobby practicing the skill with the receptionist and any children who enter the office. Additionally, the therapist might want to ask the child's parent to invite a friend of the child, or a same-age relative, to a treatment session or two to practice. A clear benefit of this approach is that the therapist can be present to give immediate feedback to the client on her use of the targeted skill(s)—something that can't be done when the child practices skills only between sessions. In essence, it is helpful to include lots of practice opportunities—either during the session or outside of treatment—to enhance learning and the generalization of the skills taught.

Individual therapy should be integrated with other forms of treatment the child may be receiving. At the most basic level, this advice means communicating with other providers in the child's life such as the psychiatrist, pediatrician, case manager, school counselor or primary teacher, and other interventionists (e.g., occupational or speech therapists). At a broader level, therapy should be integrated with the child's educational program. Assuming appropriate parental consent and assent from the child or adolescent, the therapist should specifically work with school officials to ensure that the skills being taught in therapy are supported in the classroom and that any information or feedback on inappropriate skill use or problem behaviors is communicated back to the therapist. Such communication can promote better skill use and may lead to further creative intervention strategies (e.g., changing environmental contingencies in the classroom).

In conclusion, families often seek the services of a therapist to help their son or daughter with ASD develop better social skills. In my own experience, targeting social skills development in the clinical setting is often quite challenging—not only for the reasons already discussed (e.g., poor generalization, difficulty in practicing skills with peers) but also because individual therapy typically does not have a single point focus. In other words, a key reason for referral might be to improve the child's social competence, but invariably other concerns are also highly relevant and therefore also require attention. For example, family relationships might be strained, and the child might be experiencing significant academic difficulties, both of which would distract the child during treatment and interfere with her parents' availability to practice the skills. It can be a challenge to stay focused on the target (developing the client's social competence) while attending to other salient issues in the client's life. Perhaps the two most important skills for the therapist who treats youths on the autism spectrum to possess are flexibility and empathy. The clinician needs to be flexible enough with treatment planning to adopt those approaches and strategies that best meet the client's particular needs and learning style. Second, youths with ASD face countless challenges in their daily lives: navigating confusing social situations, handling conflicts, interpreting other peoples' emotions, and understanding their own emotions and responses. Having someone they can trust, with whom they feel comfortable enough to ask personal and sometimes embarrassing questions, and with whom they can share their concerns and fears is vitally important. The therapist can be this person by being available, behaving in a trustworthy way, and demonstrating understanding and empathy.

Case Example

"Marco," a sixth-grade student with PDD-NOS, was referred for treatment by his parents for depression and suicidal ideation. He had made threats to harm himself (although he had made no actual attempts yet) as well as threats of violence against peers and teachers at school. At the clinical intake with his parents, Marco adamantly denied that there was "anything wrong" with him and said he didn't think he really had an autism spectrum disorder. Based on his school history and the parents' report, Marco was intellectually gifted and a precocious pianist. He experienced most of his difficulties in school, although his relationship with his parents was not as strong as it was when he was younger. He attended a public middle school in an affluent neighborhood and felt considerable pressure to perform academically and in sports. However, Marco struggled with problems with motor coordination. He was rather tall for his age and quite awkward physically, making it difficult for him to succeed in physical education or organized sports. Based on his parents' report, Marco had no friends at school. His teachers described him as "domineering and bossy" and stated that he was often left out of peers' activities because of the way he interacted with them.

    The incident preceding his referral occurred at school. In his English class he yelled at two peers "I'm gonna kill you!" and proceeded to throw their books and school supplies on the floor and to strike the wall with his fists before running out of the room. Reportedly the two boys, who were best friends, were just talking quietly near Marco before the eruption. Marco told his mother that the two were talking about him and saying mean things. Marco's teacher reported that, although she could not hear what the boys were saying, she doubted they were actually talking about Marco.

Individual therapy with Marco proceeded slowly at first. He needed time to feel comfortable with the therapist and often reverted to talking about daily events (e.g., his new dog or weekend plans) whenever more emotionally charged topics were brought up, such as the problems with his peers at school. By the third session, Marco was more willing to talk about his emotions and peer relationships. He recognized that his peers didn't seem to like him, but he wasn't sure why. He said they were "just mean" or "dumb." Following some therapist self-disclosure and incorporation of social vignettes and problem solving, we identified other possibilities, including the way that Marco interacted with them—for example, insisting that projects be done his way or telling others what to do—and his emotional reactivity in class. Marco eventually acknowledged that these behaviors might have an impact on peers' reactions toward him.

Once Marco understood that his behaviors might be contributing to his feelings of isolation and his lack of friends at school, he was motivated to try to do things differently. The remainder of therapy addressed two related goals: emotion regulation and cognitive restructuring. Marco worked on developing more appropriate ways to express his intense emotions—specifically, either by drawing or asking to leave class to talk to the counselor (though he agreed to talk to the counselor, at most, only once a day, a solution the school principal and nurse also agreed with). He practiced these strategies, via role play and with his parents, before using them in school. Marco also eventually identified a primary "error" in his thinking that contributed to his depressed and angry feelings, namely, his tendency to jump to conclusions. For example, in the English class incident with the two boys, Marco had automatically assumed they were talking maliciously about him because they were whispering. During several sessions, Marco worked on identifying his automatic thoughts, or cognitive errors, related to this incident and challenging them.

At the end of treatment, Marco was interacting better with his peers at school and had even been invited to a friend's house for dinner, something that had never happened before. He still struggled at times in managing his intense negative emotions, but his parents helped him by reminding him to use his coping tools or to take a break before reacting—in other words to problem-solve and cool off. He was no longer making threats of self-harm, and he reported no feelings of depression.

CHAPTER 7

Promoting Social Skills Training at Home

A child's parents or caregivers are the most powerful change agents in the child's life. No matter how much therapy a youngster is provided, the parent remains the "constant" factor as the child grows up. In most cases it is parents, followed by teachers, who spend the most time with their children. The shared goal of meeting the developmental needs of the child requires considerable interdependency and collaboration. As a consequence, cooperation between parents and teachers is crucial. Therapists and counselors are often called upon to further facilitate this collaborative process and aid parents in helping their children develop improved social skills. This chapter provides information and targeted strategies that therapists and educators can use to support parents in helping their children and teens develop age-appropriate social skills and overcome obstacles they may face.

Parent-Implemented Strategies

Parent Training

"What can we do to help him have more friends?" This is one of the questions clinicians probably hear most frequently from parents of children with ASD. Parents often want to be taught how to help their child develop his or her social skills. Most of the strategies covered in previous chapters can easily be adapted for use in the home and be implemented by the child's parents. When a clinician works directly with a child to teach social skills, it is typically helpful to also include the parent in the intervention. In some circumstances, parents may be the primary or even sole focus of the training. In other words, the professional works directly

126

with the parents, who then implement the training strategies with their child—in effect, training the trainer. Intervention provided directly to the parents rather than the child might also be advisable whenever financial constraints or other limitations (e.g., the family members can attend only a few sessions) are likely to make a child-focused intervention less feasible.

There is some evidence that parent training interventions, in which the parent is instructed by the clinician on various approaches or methods to use, are most effective when the parent can be trained in natural environments such as the family's home (Rocha, Schreibman, & Stahmer, 2007). This option, however, is not always feasible: it may be too far for the clinician to travel to the family's home, time may be a limiting factor, or the parents or clinician may feel uncomfortable with this alternative. Even if the training does not occur in the home, however, the clinician can gather detailed information about the home environment to develop interventions that best suit the family. For example, knowing that the child goes to his grandparents' house when he comes home from school because his mother doesn't get home until later in the evening is important, especially if one of the treatment objectives is identifying nearby peers to play with after school. Seeing the neighborhood in which the family lives and noting how busy the street is that the family lives on and whether or not there are similar-age children around could be valuable information. Indeed, significant indicators of a training program's success include the parent's ability to adapt the strategies to diverse environments and to prove the suitability of the chosen techniques to both the child and family as well as the particular environment.

There are many likely benefits of parent training or parent-directed intervention(s), including the following:

* Interventions implemented by parents tend to be cost-effective.
* Parent-led interventions can be more time-intensive for the child and much more continuous than other types of interventions.
* The interventions can more easily be conducted in natural settings.
* The generalization of skills to targeted settings (e.g., the home, the school) is more likely to be realized.

Incorporating Natural Teaching Methods into Everyday Family Activities

In the home, incorporating visual teaching tools and reminders into the child's training and practicing exercises can be useful. Parents can use cues (whether visual or auditory), flash cards, or cutouts (e.g., arrows, cartoons showing various facial expressions) to prompt their child about staying on topic, turn-taking, using appropriate nonverbal communication, and other conversational skills (Ozonoff, Dawson, McPartland, 2002). Of course, such stimuli should not be used continuously, or else it is likely that the child will either grow tired of them, become too dependent on them, and/or resist their use. It may be more beneficial to have "dedicated training times" built into the child's schedule during which these tools are used. A dedicated half-hour after dinner each evening to talk about and practice a new skill, for example, might readily fit into the family's schedule.

Other activities that can be used as natural social skills training opportunities include family games and meals. Many games such as hangman, charades, I-spy, or multiplayer board games can be modified to make them more social in nature. As an example, a game of I-spy might take place in the park, and the key rule would be that things that are "spied" must be related to observing the actions of other people (e.g., "I spy someone laughing," "I spy a woman with a black dog"). During a board game, before each person takes a turn, he might say one thing he learned that day or is looking forward to the next day. Or, during hangman the person at the drawing board could practice giving compliments or praise (e.g., "no 'g'—but good guess") after each person makes a guess.

At family meals, obvious social skills to practice include table manners, but attending to such conversational skills as staying on-topic could also be made a focal point. Kids often have fun with role reversal. For instance, Dad might intentionally make mistakes (such as saying something off-topic) and see if the kids can catch the error before Mom does. Videotaping some of these family activities to watch later can have the added benefit of demonstrating to the child how certain skills look and how much the child has improved in successfully demonstrating a particular skill over time. Working with a family that is implementing such a strategy, the therapist might ask that some home videos of these *in vivo* training sessions (e.g., a sit down meal, the family's game night) be brought in to the treatment sessions. The therapist can then give feedback to the child on her use of targeted skills as well as offer suggestions to the parents on ways of improving or refining their training methods and social interactions. The therapist may notice, for example, that the mother tends to take the lead in prompting the child on how to respond and that the child is subsequently becoming prompt-dependent on Mom—waiting for his cue from her about how to respond and what to do.

Locating Helpful Peers and Encouraging Appropriate Friendships

Parents can be instrumental in finding a same-age peer who is socially skilled and tolerant and with whom their child can practice new social skills. While achieving this objective is not easy, having one identified peer to "guide" the child with ASD in social interactions can make other peer interactions go much more smoothly. It is not important whether the identified peer attends the same school. In fact, some parents find it's better that they be in different schools as the child might become upset when the identified peer interacts with other students or may put pressure on the peer to choose among friends. The peer also might be put in a difficult social situation if the child with ASD does something offensive or socially objectionable and the other kids know the two are buddies. Depending on the community and what is available, some resources for parents to consider in trying to find potentially suitable friends for their child include sports leagues, extracurricular classes (e.g., martial arts), group music lessons, local recreational centers or swim clubs, or day camps. Another option for parents who work outside the home is to find colleagues with same-age children who might fit the bill. Arranging social events such as a picnic and inviting the other family can promote the development of a possible friendship for the children and possibly provide social support to the parents as well.

It is important for parents to nurture the peer relationships of the child with ASD. Parents must determine, with their child's input, how much the other child and his or her parents should be told about the ASD diagnosis. Sometimes sharing information about the spectrum disorder is necessary—particularly if, for example, it is likely that the child will overreact to minor things the peer might do or say, or perhaps become upset for no apparent reason. It is important that the relationship not be entirely orchestrated by the parents, that it not be the result of pity from the other child or his parents, or that the peer not feel or be coerced into the arrangement. Also, the parents have to be careful not to overburden the peer or appear to be buying his time or attention for their own child.

Finding or supporting social relationships is usually easier to achieve with younger children. As children get older, many resist parental involvement in determining their peer relationships—as do the peers. The parents of a young teen might simply drop occasional reminders about initiating social invitations to their son or daughter (e.g., "We don't have any family plans this weekend, so if you want to ask one of your friends to come over, that would be fine with us"), offer suggestions for activities, and/or be available to provide transportation if needed.

Purposefully Planning Social Activities and Playdates

There is empirical evidence that having typically developing friends promotes social development in preadolescent children with ASD (Bauminger et al., 2008). Identifying appropriate peer groups in which a child might form such a friendship is therefore a goal of many parents. Organizing a group of children for their son or daughter to interact with socially (Vismara, Gengoux, Boettcher, Koegel, & Koegel, 2006) can be very helpful. For youths with ASD, this objective might be most easily accomplished when there is already a group organized around a particular interest or subject mater that is also genuinely interesting to their child. For a girl who is good at and enjoys science, for example, the parent might try to find a science club or consider creating one if one doesn't already exist by working with the school's science teacher. For a child with a special interest in building robots, a family that lives near a college or university might check with the engineering or computer science departments about clubs in which the child might participate.

Of course, it is not always possible to find a club that matches exactly—or even closely—their child's unique interests. Sometimes more common social clubs such as Boy Scouts or 4-H can be suitable and helpful as an outlet for practicing social skills for children with ASD. The potential downside is that most such groups are not designed for children with ASD, and it is not the mission of these groups to "teach" social skills. To be an enjoyable and successful experience for the child, he will need explicit instruction on how to behave, what to say and do, etc., before group meetings. This requirement is also true for parent-arranged playdates. It usually takes very heavy involvement on the part of the parent to make a one-on-one social engagement successful for a child with ASD. Below I list several specific suggestions for helping to make these activities happy and productive social encounters:

- Start small—make the initial interactions relatively short events (e.g., 20–30 minutes, at most). As the children get more comfortable with one another and if things go well, gradually increase the length of the social engagements. It is more important that each encounter end on a positive note than that they be lengthy.
- Be closely involved in the activity, at least at the beginning. Parents should stay near their child in case he needs coaching or support, or runs into a problem.
- Gradually fade out the parent's involvement. With each social activity or playdate, the parent should become less and less involved in the activity. By the third time a friend comes over, for

example, the parent might stay within earshot but not be involved in the activity.

- Provide as much structure as needed, especially for initial social encounters. Arranging the activity around a particular event, such as making a pizza, can provide some parameters for assessing what is expected and how long the activity will likely take.

Parents usually need some guidance in setting up social activities for their children. Afterward, if things did not go as well as the parent had hoped for, problem solving and reviewing the suggestions listed above may uncover something that might have been overlooked (e.g., the parent set up a daylong outing when the child was by no means ready for such a lengthy activity).

Explaining the Nature of Friendships

Many young people with ASD have difficulty recognizing who their friends really are and do not understand or appreciate the reciprocal nature of genuine friendships (Bauminger et al., 2008). A young girl with ASD, for instance, might have a tendency to identify the most popular or athletic girls in school as her "best friends" even if she has never been invited to visit their homes, for example. It can be as emotionally upsetting for the parent as it is for their daughter when she is teased by someone whom she thinks is a friend. Teasing is confusing for the child and can lead to a host of other problems such as depression or aggression.

Parents can be instrumental in helping their children to learn to distinguish among friends, acquaintances, and the kids who mainly tease or bully them. The parent might begin a dialogue about friendships in an educational, matter-of-fact way. For example, a discussion about friendships might follow an age-appropriate television show that they watch together. The parent comments on things that the kids do *to* and *with* one another in the show that indicate whether they are "friends" or "nonfriends." If the child seems open to talking about this subject, the parent and child can develop a "friend chart" together (see the example in Figure 7.1). The chart needs to be created and modified to fit each child's particular needs. This activity can help the child learn which behaviors to watch for and may help him rethink whom he has been viewing as friends. The parent should first try to come up with labels for what the child naturally calls each type of person (these are usually different labels than what the parent would use). Use the child's language for labeling each type of peer (e.g., "buddy," "just someone I hang out with school," "someone I should stay away from"). Three very different

Category	What they might do ...	What I might do ...	What I should NOT do ...
Friends	Invite me over, ask what I am doing after school, sit by me at lunch	Ask how their weekend was, invite them over to my house	Don't be possessive or get upset if they have other friends, don't hog all their time
Peers	Sit by me in class but not in the lunchroom, talk to me at school	Talk to them, invite them to be involved in a group project	Don't get upset if they don't sit by me
Bullies/ nonfriends	Mock me, spread gossip, laugh at me, call me names; kick, hit, or stare at me; get others to leave me out of activities	Walk away and try to ignore it; make sure I am in a group and not alone; if they hurt me, tell a trusted adult	Don't show them that I am upset or cry; don't hit back

FIGURE 7.1. Example of a "friend chart."

types of peers that it may be helpful to distinguish clearly in the child's mind are:

- *Friend* = buddy, best friend(s), primary friend.
- *Peer/fellow student* = someone who could become a friend, classmate, or secondary friend; a kid I just hang out with at school.
- *Non-friend* = bully; someone who makes fun of me or teases me; someone I don't talk to—even in school.

The parent and child can then talk about the behaviors that each type of person is likely to exhibit. For example, a "friend" might ask you to do things with him on the weekend or after school, but a "peer" is someone you just talk to at lunch or in class. Finally, the parent and child can discuss what the child should and should not do in response to each type of person. Remember that the "do's" are just as important— perhaps even more important—than the "do not's"—so that the child knows what she should be doing when faced with any given situation. This rudimentary "friend chart" can be modified as needed to make it maximally helpful to the child. Some children like to color-code the different types of peers (e.g., friends are shaded in yellow, nonfriends in red), and may even wish to categorize the students in their class according to their chart.

True friendship requires relatively high-level social skills such as understanding and showing feelings, theory-of-mind skills, respect for individual differences, and a fair degree of empathy. Such skills are difficult to teach and typically quite difficult for people with ASD to learn. Sometimes—especially for teenagers with ASD—having one or two good friends may be more valuable than having a large group of friends. Indeed, school-age children with HFA and AS have been found to generally have fewer friends in school than peers without ASD (Wainscot, Naylor, Sutcliffe, Tantam, & Williams, 2008). This finding is important for parents to be aware of, as it may well be more worthwhile for the typical child with ASD to practice skills for continuing and maintaining existing friendships rather than striving to create a larger (and most likely less intimate) group of friends.

Helping the Child with ASD Handle Bullying

Parents often come to counselors or school professionals with questions about how they should handle reports of their child being picked on or bullied at school. In general, I suggest trying to intervene and protect the child—but not in a way that might make the bullying worse. This can be a daunting challenge. Some approaches that might inadvertently worsen the problem include talking to the teacher in front of the child's class or peers and instructing the child to "fight back. " Some helpful strategies include the following:

- Enlist school officials' help in finding a peer buddy to stay with the child during unstructured time periods, like recess and lunch, when teasing is more likely to occur.
- Talk about any specific behaviors the child is engaging in that might be contributing to the teasing. Emphasize the child's strengths and unique talents and talk about how, just because some of his behaviors are unusual, that doesn't mean he is wrong or bad. If he wants to fit in better with peers, however, he may need to modify certain behaviors so that he doesn't stand out so emphatically. This advice also applies to the child's style of dress (e.g., insisting on wearing only sweatpants instead of jeans to school), grooming, and hygiene—in short, anything that is likely to attract unwanted attention.
- Ask school personnel to keep an eye out for bullying *wherever* the child reports it happening (e.g., in lesser traveled and unsupervised areas of the playground). Ask the child specifically where and when any bullying took place so these areas can be better patrolled during the most vulnerable times of the day.
- In general, try to institute *prevention* measures wherever possible.

Modeling Social Problem Solving, Self-Talk, and Emotional Insight

Difficulty with theory-of-mind skills (inferring and understanding others' thoughts, intentions, and feelings [e.g., Baron-Cohen, 1995]) and with executive functions (monitoring one's own behaviors to achieve future goals [e.g., Ozonoff, 1997]) may underlie many of the social difficulties children with ASD experience. Parents' ability to make their thinking about their own social issues and problems *explicit and transparent*, therefore, can be a good teaching tool. In other words, very direct and explicit modeling can be very useful for some children.

Parents should consider talking through any social difficulties they are currently experiencing "out loud" with their child. Such everyday occurrences as a conflict with a coworker or having to speak publicly at the PTA meeting despite being anxious about doing so can demonstrate how the parent's own internal dialogue (i.e., that which is normally kept private) guides his or her behavior and choices. With social situations specifically, this technique can help the child appreciate the reasons for certain social behaviors (e.g., chit-chat with others while standing in line or with the cashier at the grocery store) that might not otherwise be obviously clear.

Modeling can also be helpful in developing a child's emotional insight. Parents can make comments on their own emotions and those observed in others (e.g., "He looks upset—I wonder if he just got some bad news"). I also think it is generally a good idea for parents to verbally label their own emotions even though most parents have a tendency to protectively "hide" intense or negative emotions from their children. If Mom had a bad day at work, actually *expressing* some of the details can help the child to understand why she feels so upset—and also how she plans to deal with her feelings. Briefly verbalizing one's feelings on occasion can demonstrate that it is okay to talk about bad things that happen to us and that our feelings are connected to things we experience and the ways in which we think about these things. By being proactive and taking a problem-solving approach to one's own emotions, the parent models important emotion regulation skills to the observant child.

Consider the following hypothetical example of what a mother says to her son on their way home from school: "What a day I had! My boss gave me someone else's paperwork to finish—on top of what I already have! I thought it was really unfair of him. I think I will take a long walk when we get home to cool off." The boy might not comment or offer his mother comfort or suggestions on how to handle her problem, but his mother's sharing aspects of her emotional life with him helps demonstrate that *everyone* has "bad days"—and that's when problem solving kicks in!

Common Obstacles or "Parent Traps"

Siblings: Challenges and Benefits

Typically developing siblings can be a wonderful resource in promoting skill use and generalization among those with ASD. Siblings provide natural and immediate feedback to youths with ASD, and they are usually readily available as partners in practicing new skills. Preliminary studies on the use of siblings and peers as trainers have shown promising results (e.g., Bass & Mulick, 2008; Dodd et al., 2008). On the other hand, when the sibling is considerably more socially successful, there can be challenges for both the youth with ASD and the sibling. The child with ASD may engage in an unhealthy comparison by, on first impression, contrasting his own failings and failures with his sibling's relative good fortune and popularity. Jealousy or other negative feelings can easily arise, putting additional strains on the siblings' relationship and the entire family.

For the normally functioning sibling, having a brother or sister who behaves in odd and unpredictable ways can be very challenging. It can sometimes be difficult to invite friends over to the house, and it is especially challenging when the siblings attend the same school. Siblings of children with ASD have, indeed, been found to exhibit more behavioral problems than siblings of nonaffected children or even children who have Down syndrome (Fisman, Wolf, Ellison, & Freeman, 2000). In some instances, the child with ASD may try to "tag along" with his sibling and his closest friends even when he is obviously not wanted. This dilemma quickly becomes a problem when the sibling wants to spend time with his closest friends apart from his brother or sister.

So, what can parents do when these types of situations arise between siblings? One strategy is to explain to both children that some friends are friends of both kids and some friends are one child's friend, or "not to be shared." Many youths with ASD, as already noted, struggle mightily to understand the nature of friendship. A matter-of-fact explanation such as the following can be helpful.

> "Ben is your brother's friend. They are the same age and enjoy doing things by themselves occasionally. When Ben is over at the house, he and your brother will usually want to play by themselves. They aren't trying to leave you out, but they need time just for the two of them. But you and your brother are both friends of Tim and Luke. They are our neighbors, and you can play with them together."

Reinforcing and praising the typical (non-ASD) sibling's social skills can be helpful. It can make that child feel special—an important consideration, given that so much parental attention and time is spent on addressing concerns for the sibling with ASD and arranging appropriate treatments. Also, identifying the sibling's prosocial skills and showing how important you think it is that she have such good skills can motivate her to help their brother or sister with ASD to develop better social skills. The ideal scenario is that of a typical sibling taking on the role of helper (in terms of social skills practice for the sibling with ASD) on her own initiative. If a child willingly and *independently* takes on the role of "practice partner," however, it is important that she recognize that this is not a permanent or unrelenting role. In other words, at times she is "just" a sibling and not always a junior coach to her sibling with ASD.

Parents may find it helpful to have designated times dedicated to practicing social skills. If the child with ASD is learning a certain skill, such as taking turns during games, then the parent might want to oversee some games at home between the child with ASD and the sibling (1) to observe what the child naturally tends to do, or what might get in the way of successful skill use (e.g., telling the other child what to do), and (2) to prompt use of the correct skill as needed. Some of the specific ways that siblings can help promote the learning and repeated practicing of new social skills at home include making overtures toward the sibling with ASD, encouraging speech during play activities and praising appropriate play behavior, and prompting age-appropriate initiations and responses (see Bass & Mulick, 2007, for a review).

Avoid Being Overly Directive

The poor pragmatic communications skills of children with ASD can contribute to patterns of parent–child interaction that unfortunately do not facilitate growth in the child's social communicative repertoire. For instance, the child with autism might initiate with his parent only very infrequently or do so in atypical ways. This failing can lead to a greater frequency of parent-directed discourse, more initiations by the parent, and communication that usually comes across as didactic, or too parent-directed, in nature. Parents are advised to be attentive to the social communicative attempts made by the child even when these attempts are not entirely appropriate or clear. Responding to them can help to increase the child's initiations and communications with their parents or other adults in the future. Using child-focused language and closely attending to the pragmatics of communication (rather than a style that is parent-directed or in which the parent controls the interaction) can be helpful. Consider the differences in the following examples of parent–child verbal interactions:

Parent-directed

• "Go get the truck to play with!"
• "Let's play chess."

Child-focused

• "You brought me your cup. Do you want more juice?"
• "You have the red truck, so I will be the green truck—should we race?"

There is a substantial body of research on parent-mediated interventions to promote appropriate language use and communication, a thorough review of which is beyond the scope of this chapter (see Aldred, Pollard, Phillips, & Adams, 2001; Aldred, Green, & Adams, 2004). For parents, adapting communication patterns to meet the child's needs while reinforcing the child's attempts at interaction can promote social engagement and reciprocity.

It's Never Too Early to Think Ahead

There is considerable variability in outcomes among adults with ASD. Some people are able to complete degrees in the field of their choice, marry and have families, and maintain gainful employment. Unfortunately, however, the quality of adult outcomes is usually not commensurate with that seen in non-ASD peers—even for higher-functioning people on the spectrum. Some of the difficulties commonly seen are continued dependence on families and parents, low employment status, a lack of close friends, and not having life partners or spouses (Howlin, Goode, Hutton, & Rutter, 2004; Engstrom, Ekstrom, & Emilsson, 2003). Both previous research and my own clinical experience suggest that many young adults with ASD are socially isolated, lonely, and possibly depressed. They face many challenges, including difficulties in achieving an independent lifestyle, unsatisfactory employment circumstances, and a general lack of social support.

Why are adult outcomes so variable and often poorer than expected? Problems with multitasking, time management, and planning ahead (i.e., executive function deficits) can make it difficult to succeed in college or to live independently. Deficits with social reciprocity and emotional insight can make the prospects of maintaining long-term friendships, dating, and eventually marriage dubious. For parents, planning ahead for transitions (into middle school and high school, and then out of formal education into independent living) can be helpful. The following suggestions can be applied to social skills development but may apply to other areas of the child's life as well:

- Parents should talk to their child's school and education team (if applicable) about transition planning early. Try to plan at least 1 year in advance for upcoming transitions.
- Try to identify someone who can "coach" the child on life skills, such as filling out job applications or obtaining a driver's permit. It can be easier sometimes if this person is not a parent (to promote separation and independence) but perhaps a family member your child looks up to, a counselor, or an involved teacher.
- Investigate support groups for teens or young adults with ASD in your locality. If one doesn't exist, the parents should consider trying to start one by talking to local counselors or therapists who work with people with ASD about participating in and helping to organize one.
- Some parents encourage their child to consider community college close to home before attempting to transition to a larger university or to complete independent living, to make the transition more gradual.
- Teach the child self-sufficiency skills (e.g., answering the telephone, setting up appointments), and, with improved competence, build on these skills by allowing the child to take on more complex tasks.

Case Example

"Charlie's" parents knew they had to do something about his poor social skills at mealtimes. Charlie, an 8-year-old, was diagnosed with high-functioning autism. He attended a regular-education public elementary school, and at least once a week his parents got reports from school officials that Charlie had gotten into another fight with a peer at lunch. Invariably, each incident appeared to be instigated by inappropriate behavior on Charlie's part.

Charlie would chew with his mouth open and talk continuously while eating. He would also invade peers' and siblings' physical space—often reaching onto their plates if he saw something he wanted to eat or taking their drink. At school, his classmates generally avoided sitting with him, but Charlie did not readily pick up on this. He would squeeze in between two peers sitting close together even when empty seats were available at other tables. These issues—poor personal space boundaries, not picking up on the nonverbal cues of others, and poor etiquette at meals—were also evident at home. Charlie's brothers hated eating with him. They often begged their parents to let them eat in the family room instead of with Charlie.

To help Charlie improve his social skills at mealtimes, Charlie's Mom and Dad decided to first teach appropriate social skills related to eating in a one-on-one setting. After school, Charlie's Mom would work with him for about 20 minutes (during his after-school snack) on eating with his mouth closed, taking turns while talking, and respecting each other's body space. She found a couple of movie clips showing children eating together that demonstrated these skills, which Charlie enjoyed watching, and they talked together about what they saw.

When Charlie and his mom thought he was ready, he practiced these skills during family dinners with his brothers. His parents videotaped the meals, and family members watched clips of the videos as a group in the evenings, talking about what things went right and what things could be improved. Charlie's parents were careful to point out things that the other children could improve on that were related to their own mealtime manners, not just Charlie's. After several practice meals with the family, Charlie's Dad set up a playdate with another boy in Charlie's after-school social skills group and arranged to take the two boys out to get pizza. Charlie's father coached him beforehand on what to do and not do and praised his appropriate use of the skills they had worked on. Over time, Charlie's parents became less and less involved in these arranged playdates, and they also began receiving fewer notes at home from the school officials about Charlie's difficulties at lunchtime.

CHAPTER 8

Improving Social Competence beyond Childhood

Several specific approaches and strategies for improving the social competence of youths and teenagers with ASD have been covered in this book. Regardless of the type(s) of intervention, the ASD subtype, or even the specific social challenges faced by the child, every family must make certain decisions related to the social development of their child with ASD. These decisions inevitably impact longer-term outcomes. In this final chapter, we take a look ahead to life beyond childhood for people with ASD in relation to social skills training and social competence by addressing issues related to the level of parents' involvement, peer groups and social relationships, and planning for the future.

Parents' Involvement: Changing Needs

The importance of having the child's parents closely involved in his or her social skills programming and training has been emphasized throughout this volume. Indeed, parents' support and coaching are crucial to the success of any intervention. A much less often discussed topic is how parental involvement should *change* as the child gets older. The extent and type of parental involvement differ at various stages in a child's life—or at least they *should*. With typically developing children, parents normally cease to be heavily involved in their children's peer social networks beginning in middle childhood and on into adolescence. While they maintain some interest and provide some monitoring, they generally don't schedule activities or supervise peer interactions, for instance. *Parents of children with ASD, however—painfully aware that their son's or daughter's poor skills constantly create socially awkward and often embarrassing situations—naturally wish to protect and guide them for as long as possible.* Problems arise when the child's normal desire for separation from parents and greater independence increase during later childhood or early adolescence. At that juncture, the child's greater need for independence clashes with the parents' need to protect him or her.

The families that weather this transition best are those in which the parents accept their child's growing need to be their own person. Either extreme of parental involvement—doting fretfully over the youth beyond the point where it is called for versus pushing the teen toward more independence than he or she is actually ready for—is not ideal. The mother who still carefully selects her 15-year-old son's clothes each morning (when he is quite capable of picking out his own clothes) is actually preventing him from learning an important lesson in self-care. A more age-appropriate approach that would still support the teenager and prevent him from choosing inappropriate clothing might be to designate several dresser drawers that contain clothes appropriate for school, with the bottom drawer reserved only for weekend (i.e., not appropriate for school) clothes. In sorting his laundry, he could then refresh his own memory as to which drawer was appropriate to which clothes.

Much "overparenting" also occurs in respect to scheduling and canceling appointments. With teenagers and sometimes with younger children (tweens), the therapist might request that the youth call the office if an appointment needs to be changed or cancelled or to phone him directly to let him know how a planned activity went rather than relying on the parent to do so. This invitation to more frequent communications demonstrates that the therapist believes that the youth is ready for such tasks and encourages the youth to practice an important social skill, namely, using the telephone appropriately to either report results or arrange appointments. In general, parents should continue to be available to the teenager whenever called upon for help, which usually represents a good middle-of-the-road position.

Parents themselves can sometimes benefit from the counseling that a therapist offers as their teenager makes the transition toward greater independence. Parents can express their concerns and worries to the therapist, and the teen has someone with whom she can discuss personal or social problems. In my own experience counseling preteens and adolescents with ASD, I have found it helpful to be transparent with the parents and the young client about the nature of the counseling relationship, and I explain the role that I will play from the start of the therapeutic relationship. Specifically, I make sure that the youth and parents both understand that the child (or teen) is my main client; I clarify the nature of confidentiality so that the teen trusts that she can talk about personally sensitive topics with me without her parents necessarily being privy; and I reiterate what the limits of confidentiality are and when things have to be shared with the parent (in cases of potential self-harm). With regard to this last part—what is shared with parents and the limits of confidentiality—the parents do maintain legal rights with respect to their child's therapy when the child is a minor. However, most parents understand that the youth's ability to maintain privacy in therapy affects his willingness to open up to the therapist, which is highly beneficial if not absolutely critical to treatment progress. That being so, most parents do not press for more information than what their child is inclined to convey. If a parent does press confidentiality bounds unduly, it is important that the therapist determine why. What exactly do the parents want to know or believe they need to know? Most parents want the best for their children, and being apprized of everything they need to know about the nature of the therapeutic relationship early on should help them to establish the trust they need to have in the therapist and his or her competence.

Depending on the age and maturity of the child or adolescent, I usually prefer to have the youth present when the parents are brought into sessions for progress updates or check-ins. Ideally, the youth summarizes the session content for the parent. This procedure is not always possible, however. Some youngsters are unable to synthesize what was discussed or adequately verbalize it for the parent. In such circumstances, I generally prompt the child to share certain things that are relevant from the session (e.g., "Can you tell your Mom about the practice exercise we performed today?") and if there is anything that the child misses, I ask if it is okay with him or her for me to share it with the parent(s).

Finally, understanding and accepting the child's level of need or desire for social relationships is crucially important. We know that many children with ASD would prefer more friendships and that they generally experience considerable loneliness (Bauminger & Kasari, 2000). Based on clinical observations and anecdotal reports, however, some children with ASD do not place as much importance on having a broad social network as non-ASD children typically do—or as much as their parents would hope. Their ideal friendships may be based on shared interests and activities (having a playmate, someone who likes the same video games) more so than emotional support and sharing (e.g., Kelly et al., 2008). It is impossible to generalize about all children with ASD with respect to their relative desire for friendships and what type of friendship they want most. Parents and clinicians both need to be aware of the potential mismatch between what the child wants and what parents think is normal, and they should be wary of assuming that their social ambitions map well onto those of a child with ASD.

The therapist can usually get an idea of the child's social goals and interests via an in-depth intake interview—by finding out what types of things make the child happy (e.g., social things?), what things in her life bother her or she wishes were different, and what she generally thinks of other kids her age. Of course, this type of information is harder to gather from a very young child, in which case behavioral observations may be informative—noting, for instance, whether the child seems to be interested in and readily observes peers or rather is wary of them, aloof, and inclined to disregard others' approaches. It is also worth noting that some older children deny loneliness or a desire for more friends and yet exhibit behaviors that indicate otherwise. One young man I worked with, for example, claimed to have no interest in making friends with people in his high school. Yet, he spent a great deal of time in internet chat rooms and greatly enjoyed "speaking" to people online. When he obtained a part-time job at a music store, he was clearly happy that he was meeting people of his own age, most of whom did not attend his school. In this circumstance, it appeared that the youth did actually want and enjoy social interaction but was uneasy about talking to people in his school.

Peer Groups: New and Old

Parents and educators have strong feelings about whether or not to disclose that a student has an ASD to peers. On the one hand, there is concern about widespread negative publicity about people with autism and the potential for stigmatizing attitudes and behaviors. On the other hand, disclosure may promote better communication and improve peers' attitudes. The debate about ASD disclosure is far from settled, and, in the end, it is a choice that the parents, child or teen, and school officials should make together. For a comprehensive review of the factors one should consider before disclosing ASD to peers, see Campbell (2006). Specific strategies for promoting successful integration of those with ASD and typically developing students in school are provided in the volumes by Harrower and Dunlap (2001) and Williams, Johnson, and Sukhodolsky (2005).

As described by Williams and colleagues (2005), methods for promoting social integration within inclusive classrooms include antecedent-based strategies, peer-mediated strategies, and directive skills training approaches. Examples of antecedent-based strategies include incorporation of multiple group-learning activities and projects and teacher modeling of prosocial skills. Training peers on how to interact with a student with ASD and buddy programs are examples of peer-mediated approaches. As earlier discussed at length in Chapter 5, social skills training delivered in the school setting has many benefits, including the ready availability of peers with whom to practice and a learning environment that matches the actual targeted environment where it is hoped the skills will be utilized (Williams et al., 2005). Additional benefits of receiving training in the school include the fact that the intervention may be at no cost (or reduced cost) to parents, potentially avoiding scheduling and transportation difficulties—which is especially important for families with limited resources—and it can fulfill important educational mandates if improved social competence is targeted among a child's IEP objectives.

One of the main frustrations that I hear from parents and from the children with ASD themselves relates to the way that peers view them and treat them. It is an unfortunate reality that, for most kids, the peer group's attitude will not change very much—*regardless of how much better the child's social skills become!* For many children with ASD, this circumstance means that they have to stay with much the same group of peers that has seen them run out of the classroom in tears because they didn't know how to answer a question, behave inappropriately in the lunchroom, or possibly even be escorted out of the school by the principal or a policeman following aggressive threats. In other words, children on the autism spectrum might learn new skills and be able to interact with peers, but previous negative social experiences—and the collective social memory among the peer group—might continue to follow them.

For some children, it can be most helpful to just find a new peer group. This alternative does not necessarily mean changing schools completely (though this can sometimes be the best option) but more often means finding a different activity or social outlet that will afford the child new opportunities to make friends with same-age peers. Some possibilities to consider include youth activity groups (e.g., 4-H Club, Boy or Girl Scouts), special camps, after-school organizations, special-interest clubs, and church youth groups. Keep in mind that it can also be a relief for many children to enter middle school from elementary school or high school from middle school. Such transitions can rightly be regarded as "fresh starts" and are often accompanied by opportunities to meet many new people. The change can be anxiety provoking, but it can also be treated as a welcome chance to meet new kids who will also be starting something new.

Planning for the Future

Autism and the other spectrum disorders are usually lifelong conditions. Yet, there is tremendous variability in terms of outcomes for adults with ASD. The factors that appear to most affect eventual outcomes and one's degree of independence are the cognitive functioning level (Cederlund, Hagberg, Billstedt, Hillberg, & Gillberg, 2008) and—particularly—

verbal ability (Eaves & Ho, 2008). Even among cognitively high-functioning individuals, however, adult outcomes are typically not commensurate with those seen in non-ASD peers. In other words, a person's independence and quality of life may not correspond with what would be predicted based on cognitive functioning alone. Often, people with ASD report having very few close friends or partners, being too dependent on their families, and having low employment status or lacking gainful employment (Howlin et al., 2004; Engstrom et al., 2003).

There is certainly no easy solution for how best to plan for the future to increase the chances of social success in adulthood. However, especially for higher-functioning youths, it is probably important to educate them fully about their particular disorder(s) and the enduring nature of the social challenges associated with ASD. Acceptance of the diagnosis, including associated strengths as well as deficits, can help to reduce stigma and make the individual more willing to seek and therefore receive help in the future. Explaining to an adolescent that social relationships will probably always be challenging can be a difficult thing to do. But doing so can help prevent or at least lessen later disappointment and frustration. Related to this approach, identifying realistic and attainable goals for social development can be quite motivating. A child should have short-term goals—such as talking to someone new at camp within the next 2 weeks—as well as longer-term goals—for instance, inviting someone out on a date. As the adolescent matures, new goals related to growing independence need to be set (e.g., taking the test for a driver's permit, applying for a part-time job). Setbacks are inevitable; it is how the child and family handle them that really affects ultimate improvement and outcomes.

Other suggestions for long-term planning, especially for transitions, include identifying a "support person"—usually someone outside the immediate family. This person might be a therapist or informal counselor or perhaps even an uncle who lives nearby, as long as it is someone with whom the youth feels comfortable. A support person might be viewed as being akin to a "coach"—a person who doesn't do things *for* the youth but, rather, guides him on *how* to accomplish his goals and provides encouragement. The support person can give advice to the youth on social concerns (e.g., dating), help her with filling out school or job applications, advocate for her and with her as needed, and generally be available should the youth have a problem she needs help with. Therapists who work with children with ASD often maintain contact with the families after the active phase of therapy or the intervention ends. The child may come in for "booster" sessions as needed, or the parents may seek consultation on handling certain transitions or challenges within the family.

In the next generation of research in the field of ASD, there will be a growing need to develop and evaluate appropriate interventions and supports for young adults. Colleges and universities, for instance, are faced with a growing number of incoming students each year who have identified autism spectrum disorders. There is unfortunately very little guidance for practitioners who work with adults or for university administrators on how to effectively help these students succeed and reach their potential.

Parents, educators, and practitioners can be instrumental in this endeavor as advocates for young people who have ASD by informing applied research and assisting in these transitions. A parent sharing with the university's student disability office her knowledge about her son's unique challenges and what has helped him in the past is invaluable. The student's past teachers might compile information about what has helped him learn, what accommodations have been found to be most useful, and how he has managed social relationships at school, all of which could be assembled into a portfolio for the parents or the young man to keep and share with his professors and counselor or academic coach. Additionally, if he has been seeing a therapist regularly, this person might offer to help the youth find a new therapist on his campus and relay pertinent information to that person.

When parents ask, as they almost inevitably will, "What can I expect long-term for my son or daughter?", the obvious answer is "It depends". It depends on a host of factors, including the child's overall functioning, cognitive and verbal abilities, social motivations and interests, the extent of interfering behaviors, and the relative self-sufficiency or level of independence—just to name a few relevant factors. But this answer is not terribly helpful, nor is it very hopeful. *Yes—it depends*, but what may be more helpful is for the practitioner to share with the parents a realistic range of possible outcomes. We know that intervention can help many children with ASD improve their social functioning. We also know that ASD is, in most cases, lifelong. As such, having short-term objectives and realistic long-term goals is advisable. Helping the youth identify his or her strengths and perhaps meet peers with ASD can be helpful. Support and education for the parents, in the form of individual counseling or a support group, can be useful as well.

Social difficulties are not exclusive to autism and other spectrum disorders, nor are they the only problem faced by youths with ASD. Deficits in social competence, nonetheless, constitute the core deficit common to all the spectrum disorders. They cut across the specific diagnostic categories as well as cognitive and language ability levels. Scientists and practitioners, at this time, are well aware that these deficits do not automatically remit with development alone; yet, we don't know the "best" approaches for intervention. Furthermore, it is highly unlikely that a single intervention approach will be ideal for all individuals with ASD.

Therefore, it is advisable to consider a variety of intervention options when targeting social skills development for a child with ASD. In treatment planning, consideration must be given to the research (e.g., what studies on the intervention have shown or the evidence for or against its use), the costs (e.g., the time needed to apply the intervention and the monetary outlays), and the fit (e.g., how likely it is that the client will find the intervention acceptable and that it will work for the client and his or her family).

As treatment progresses, evaluation should continue. Parents and practitioners must monitor progress and make changes to the treatment program as needed. It is during this monitoring process that some of the issues brought up in this chapter—the ideal degree of parental involvement, the long-term impacts on family relationships, and the nature of the ideal peer group—usually arise. Although most social skills interventions are designed for a particular child, by its very nature the ability to be socially competent relies on a number of other variables, including opportunities for appropriate social interaction, the responses the youth gets from peers and adults, and his or her perceptions of and reactions to failure and success in practicing new skills. These considerations relate to promoting the *efficacy* of the intervention, the likelihood that the learned skills will be *used* when most needed—in natural settings such as the school—and that they will be *maintained* after the active intervention ends.

APPENDIX

Reproducible Forms

Functional Assessment of Social Skills Deficits

Date and time	Child's behavior (Described in observable, measurable terms)	Antecedent (What was happening right beforehand?)	Consequence (What followed, including parent/sibling reactions?)	Any effects on family functioning? (Your thoughts on what caused or maintained the anxiety)

Social History Interview

Does the client have a best friend? _____ Yes _____ No

A group of friends? _____ Yes _____ No

    If yes, are the friends of similar age to the client? _____

    _____

    What do they do together? _____

    _____

    How often do they get together? _____

    _____

    Who coordinates gatherings? _____

    _____

How interested is the client in socializing with or making friends? Is the client motivated to improve his or her social skills?

_____

_____

_____

Describe the client's social interactions with peers (e.g., approach skills, responding to the approaches of others, eye contact, inappropriate touching or aggression):

_____

_____

_____

Does the client answer the telephone or call others? _____

_____

Any interest/involvement in electronic or virtual social networks (e.g., MySpace, Facebook, other)? _____

_____

Interest/involvement in romantic relationships or dating?

_____

_____

(cont.)

Any concerns about peer teasing/rejection?

_____

_____

_____

Any specific behaviors/vocalizations that impede social functioning?

_____

_____

_____

How does the client primarily communicate with others (e.g., in sentences? integration of nonverbal communication should be noted)? _____

_____

Has the client's hearing been tested? (if so, date) _____ Results _____

    Any concerns about hearing/perception? _____

Please describe any concerns or peculiarities regarding the client's speech (e.g., unusual pitch, volume, pace). Are the peculiarities noticeable to peers or others?

_____

_____

_____

What are your primary concerns related to the client's social functioning?

    Parent: _____

    Client: _____

153

Case Conceptualization

Name:

Parent(s):

Age:

Contact Information:

Diagnoses (*based on all available data*):

Axis I

Axis II

Axis III

Axis IV

Axis V

Social Skills Concerns (*in order, from most severe; based on observation, clinical interview, other assessments*):

1.

2.

3.

4.

Primary Social Skills Deficits (*parent report*):

1.

2.

Primary Social Skills Deficits (*child report*):

1.

2.

(*cont.*)

Case Conceptualization *(page 2 of 2)*

Selected Social Skills Target(s) (one or two, to be targeted initially in treatment):

Hypotheses about Causal and Maintaining Factors (observations, parent reports, assessment results):

Intervention Strategies:

Monitoring Plan (methods of assessment to be used and frequency of assessment):

Strengths/Interests of Client:

Potential Barriers to Treatment and Solutions:

Functional Assessment for a Child Following Two Group Sessions

Child: _____ Age: _____

Social skills concerns/goals of parent/caregiver: _____

Social skills concerns/goals of child: _____

Observations of the child during group sessions (e.g., likes, dislikes, interests, strengths, deficits): _____

SOCIAL SKILL TARGETS:

Skill/behavior	Teaching strategy to be used	Strategies for at-home practice	Rewards/other considerations

(cont.)

Functional Assessment for a Child Following Two Group Sessions *(page 2 of 2)*

BEHAVIORS THAT INTERFERE WITH APPROPRIATE SOCIALIZATION:

Behavior/concern	Antecedents (precedes, prompts behavior)	Consequences (follows, reinforces behavior)	Possible intervention/teaching strategies

Modified Functional Assessment for Student's Use

WHAT is the problem? _____

WHEN is it most likely to occur?	
WHERE is it most likely to occur?	
In what SITUATIONS is it most likely to occur?	
BEFORE it happens .. (antecedents)	
AFTER it happens ... (consequences)	

Possible hypotheses to explain this problem or behavior: _____

_____

_____

_____

What is one thing I might do to improve the social skill or behavior? _____

_____

_____

_____

ASD Psychoeducation

Here are some commonly seen attributes of people who have autism spectrum disorders. Circle any that you think apply to you, and cross out any that you think *don't* apply to you.

Honest	Loyal
Unique	Hard time with change
Rigid	Friendly
Rule-bound	Helpful
Isolated	Gullible
Alone	Emotional
Smart	Lonely
Expert	Nervous
Attentive to details	Odd
Dedicated friend	Good student

FORM 7

Goals Worksheet

Everyone has things that they are quite good at or really enjoy doing—and other things that they don't like so much or struggle with. Below we will take some time to write down some of these things.

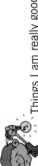 Things I am really good at (SOCIAL STRENGTHS):

Things I struggle with (SOCIAL NEEDS/DEFICITS):

Social difficulties get in the way of . . .	When I have learned and practiced some *new social skills*, I will be able to . . .

Two social goals I have: 1. _____

                              2. _____

160

Distinguishing among Thoughts, Feelings, and Actions

Thoughts are things we tell ourselves about things or people. Some examples of thoughts I have:

_____

_____

_____

Any special way I can remember how to distinguish a thought?

_____

_____

Feelings are emotions that can be felt throughout my body. Some examples of feelings I have:

_____

_____

_____

Any special way I can remember how to distinguish a feeling?

_____

_____

Actions are the things our bodies do when we have thoughts *and* feelings. Some examples of actions I do:

_____

_____

_____

Any special way I can remember how to distinguish an action?

_____

_____

Investigating Thoughts Worksheet

Thought to investigate:

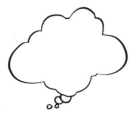

How much do you believe this thought or belief to be true and accurate? Rate it below, with *0 being completely untrue* and *100 being absolutely, without a doubt, true and accurate.*

Rating: _____

Now it is time to look at the evidence for and the evidence against this thought. *When doing the investigation, try to answer such questions as: Has this happened in the past? Does this happen to other people? Are there any other explanations?*

Evidence supporting:	Evidence not supporting:

Considering all the evidence *for* and *against* this thought/belief, make another rating of how much you believe the thought to be true and accurate.

New rating: _____

If you lowered your rating at all, try to pick which cognitive distortion is most likely at work:

_____

Problem-Solving Worksheet

1. What is the **problem?**

_____

_____

2. What is your **goal**?

_____

_____

3. What are your **reactions** (physical sensations, feelings)?

_____

_____

_____

4. What **thoughts** are you having?

5. A more **helpful thought** for solving this problem: _____

_____

_____

6. Develop a **strategy**: _____

_____

_____

7. **Evaluate**: How did you do? Time to reward your hard work!!

_____

_____

Further Reading

Resources on Inclusive Education and School-Based Strategies

Gray, C. (2000). *The new Social Story book: Illustrated edition.* Arlington, TX: Future Horizons.

Gray Center website. Provides information on Social Stories and social understanding in individuals with ASD. *www.thegraycenter.org*

Howley, M. & Arnold, E. (2005). *Revealing the hidden social code: Social Stories for people with autistic spectrum disorders.* London: Jessica Kingsley.

McConnell, K. & Ryser, G. R. (2005). *Practical ideas that really work for students with Asperger syndrome.* Austin, TX: Pro-Ed.

Williams, S. K., Johnson, C., & Sukhodolsky, D. G. (2005). The role of the school psychologist in the inclusive education of school-age children with autism spectrum disorders. *Journal of School Psychology, 43,* 117–136.

Resources for Parents and Families

Bolick, T. (2001). *Asperger syndrome and adolescence: Helping preteens and teens get ready for the real world.* Gloucester, MA: Fair Winds Press.

Jackson, L. (2002). *Freaks, geeks and Asperger syndrome: A user guide to adolescence.* London: Jessica Kingsley.

Ozonoff, S., Dawson, G., & McPartland, J. (2002). *A parent's guide to Asperger syndrome and high-functioning autism: How to meet the challenges and help your child thrive.* New York: Guilford Press.

Vismara, L. A., Gengoux, G. W., Boettcher, M., Koegel, R. L., & Koegel, L. K. (2006). *Facilitating play dates for children with autism and typically developing peers in natural settings: A training manual.* Santa Barbara: University of California Press.

Willey, L. H. (1999). *Pretending to be normal: Living with Asperger's syndrome:* London: Jessica Kingsley.

Curricula for Social Skills Instruction for Youths with ASD

Baker, J. (2003). *Social skills training for children and adolescents with Asperger syndrome and social-communication problems.* Shawnee Mission, KS: Autism Asperger Publishing.

Bellini, S. (2008). *Building social relationships: A systematic approach to teaching social interaction skills to children and adolescents with autism spectrum disorders and other social difficulties.* Shawnee Mission, KS: Autism Asperger Publishing.

McAfee, J. (2002). *Navigating the social world: A curriculum for individuals with Asperger's syndrome, high functioning autism and related disorders.* Arlington, TX: Future Horizons.

References

Aldred, C., Green, J., & Adams, C. (2004). A new social communication intervention for children with autism: Pilot randomized controlled treatment study suggesting effectiveness. *Journal of Child Psychology and Psychiatry, 45,* 1420–1430.

Aldred, C. R., Pollard, C., Phillips, R., & Adams, C. (2001). Multi-disciplinary social communication intervention for children with autism and Pervasive Developmental Disorders: The Child's Talk research project. *Journal of Educational and Child Psychology, 18,* 76–87.

American Psychiatric Association. (2000). *Diagnostic and statistical manual of mental disorders* (4th ed., text rev.). Washington, DC: Author.

Attwood, T. (2000). Strategies for improving the social integration of children with Asperger syndrome. *Autism, 4,* 85–100.

Attwood, T. (2004). Cognitive behaviour therapy for children and adults with Aperger's syndrome. *Behaviour Change, 21,* 147–161.

Bandura, A. (1994). Self-efficacy. In V. S. Ramachaudran (Ed.), *Encyclopedia of human behavior* (Vol. 4, pp. 71–81). New York: Academic Press. (Reprinted in Friedman, H. [Ed.]. [1998]. *Encyclopedia of mental health.* San Diego: Academic Press).

Barnhill, G. P., Cook, K. T., Tebbenkamp, K., & Myles, B. S.(2002). The effectiveness of social skills intervention targeting nonverbal communication for adolescents with Asperger syndrome and related pervasive developmental delays. *Focus on Autism and Other Developmental Disabilities, 17*(2), 112–118.

Baron-Cohen, S. (1995). *Mindblindness: An essay on autism and theory.* Cambridge, MA: MIT Press.

Baron-Cohen, S. (2009, November 10). The short life of a diagnosis. *The New York Times,* p. 35.

Barry, T. D., Klinger L. G., Lee J. M., Palardy N., Gilmore T., & Bodin S. D. (2003). Examining the effectiveness of an outpatient clinic-based social skills group for high-functioning children with autism. *Journal of Autism and Developmental Disorders, 33,* 685–701.

Bass, J. D., & Mulick, J. A. (2007). Social play skill enhancement of children with autism using peers and siblings as therapists. *Psychology in the Schools, 44*, 727–735.

Bauminger, N. (2007). Brief report: Group social–multimodal intervention for HFASD. *Journal of Autism and Developmental Disorders, 37*, 1605–1615.

Bauminger, N., & Kasari, C. (2000). Loneliness and friendship in high-functioning children with autism. *Child Development, 71*, 447–456.

Bauminger, N. (2002). The facilitation of social-emotional understanding and social interaction in high-functioning children with autism: Intervention outcomes. *Journal of Autism and Developmental Disorders, 32*(4), 283–298.

Bauminger, N., Shulman, C., & Agam, G. (2003). Peer interaction and loneliness in high-functioning children with autism. *Journal of Autism and Developmental Disorders, 33*(5), 489–507.

Bauminger, N., Solomon, M., Aviezer, A., Heung, K., Brown, J., & Rogers, S. J. (2008). Friendship in high-functioning children with autism spectrum disorder: Mixed and non-mixed dyads. *Journal of Autism and Developmental Disorders, 38*, 1211–1229.

Bellini, S., & Akullian, J. (2007). A meta-analysis of video modeling and video self-modeling interventions for children and adolescents with autism spectrum disorders. *Exceptional Children, 73*(3), 264–287.

Bellini, S., & Hopf, A. (2007). The development of the Autism Social Skills Profile: A preliminary analysis of psychometric properties. *Focus on Autism and Other Developmental Disabilities, 22*(2), 80–87.

Bellini, S., Peters, J. K., Benner, L., & Hopf, A. (2007). A meta-analysis of school-based social skills interventions for children with autism spectrum disorders. *Remedial and Special Education, 28*(3), 153–162.

Bogels, S. M., & Voncken, M. (2008). Social skills training versus cognitive therapy for social anxiety disorder characterized by fear of blushing, trembling, or sweating. *International Journal of Cognitive Therapy, 1*(2), 138–150.

Brown, W. H., Odom, S. L., & Conroy, M. A. (2001). An intervention hierarchy for promoting young children's peer interactions in natural environments. *Topics in Early Childhood Special Education, 21*, 162–175.

Campbell, J. M. (2006). Changing children's attitudes toward autism: A process of persuasive communication. *Journal of Developmental and Physical Disabilities, 18*, 251–272.

Campbell, J. M., Ferguson, J. E., Herzinger, C. V., Jackson, J. N., & Marino, C. A. (2004). Combined descriptive and explanatory information improves peers' perceptions of autism. *Research in Developmental Disabilities, 25*, 321–339.

Carter, A., Davis, N., Klin, A., & Volkmar, F. (2005). Social development in autism. In F. R. Volkmar, R. Paul, A. Klin, & D. Cohen (Eds.), *Handbook of autism and pervasive developmental disorders* (3rd ed., pp. 312–334). Hoboken, NJ: Wiley.

Cederlund, M., Hagberg, B., Billstedt, E., Hillberg, I. C., & Gillberg, C. (2008).

Asperger syndrome and autism: A comparative longitudinal follow-up study more than 5 years after original diagnosis. *Journal of Autism and Developmental Disorders, 38*, 72–85.

Centers for Disease Control and Prevention. (2007). Prevalence of autism spectrum disorders: Autism and Developmental Disabilities Monitoring Network. *MMWR Surveillance Summaries, 56*(1), 1–40.

Centers for Disease Control and Prevention. (2009). Prevalence of autism spectrum disorders—Autism and Developmental Disabilities Monitoring Network, United States, 2006. *MMWR Surveillance Summaries, 58*(10), 1–20.

Chalfant, A., Rapee, R., & Carroll, L. (2007). Treating anxiety disorders in children with high functioning autism spectrum disorders: A controlled trial. *Journal of Autism and Developmental Disorders, 37*, 1842–1857.

Chamberlain, B. O. (2002). Isolation or involvement?: The social networks of children with autism included in regular education classes. *Dissertation Abstracts International, 62*, 8-A, (AAI3024149).

Constantino, J. N., & Gruber, C. P. (2005). *Social Responsiveness Scale (SRS)*. Los Angeles, Western Psychological Services.

Dahle, K. B. (2003). Services to include young children with autism in the general curriculum. *Early Childhood Education Journal, 31*, 65–70.

Dawson, G. (2009). Early behavioral intervention, brain plasticity, and the prevention of autism spectrum disorder. *Development and Psychopathology, 20*, 775–803.

de Boo, G. M., & Prins, P. J. M. (2007). Social incompetence in children with ADHD: Possible moderators and mediators in social-skills training. *Clinical Psychology Review, 27*(1), 78–97.

Dodd, S., Hupp, S. D. A., Jewell, J. D., & Krohn, E. (2008). Using parents and siblings during a Social Story intervention for two children diagnosed with PDD-NOS. *Journal of Developmental and Physical Disabilities, 20*, 217–229.

Dossetor, D. R. (2007). All that glitters is not gold: Misdiagnosis of psychosis in pervasive developmental disorders—a case series. *Clinical Child Psychology and Psychiatry, 12*, 537–548.

Eaves, L.C., & Ho, H. H. (2008). Young adult outcome of autism spectrum disorders. *Journal of Autism and Developmental Disorders, 38*, 739–747.

Engstrom, I., Ekstrom, L., & Emilsson, B. (2003). Psychosocial functioning in a group of Swedish adults with asperger syndrome of high-functioning autism. *Autism, 7*, 99–110.

Evans, S. W., Axelrod, J. L., & Sapia, J. L. (2000). Effective school-based mental health interventions: Advancing the social skills training paradigm. *Journal of School Health, 70*, 191–193.

Fisman, S., Wolf, L., Ellison, D., & Freeman, T. (2000). A longitudinal study of siblings of children with chronic disabilities. *Canadian Journal of Psychiatry, 45*, 369–381.

Frith, U. (2003). *Autism: Explaining the enigma* (2nd ed.), Malden, MA: Blackwell.

Gabriels, R. L., & van Bourgondien, M. E. (2007). Sexuality and autism:

Individual, family, and community perspectives and interventions. In R. L. Gabriels & M. E. van Bourgondien (Eds.), *Growing up with autism: Working with school-age children and adolescents* (pp. 58–72). New York: Guilford Press.

Gadow, K. D., Devincent, C. J., & Drabick, D. A. G. (2008). Oppositional defiant disorder as a clinical phenotype in children with autism spectrum disorder. *Journal of Autism And Developmental Disorders, 38*(7), 1302–1310.

Gaus, V. L. (2007). *Cognitive-behavioral therapy for adult Asperger syndrome.* New York: Guilford Press.

Ghaziuddin, M. (2008). Defining the behavioral phenotype of Asperger syndrome. *Journal of Autism and Developmental Disorders, 38*(1), 138–142.

Ghaziuddin, M., Weidmar-Mikhail, E., Ghaziuddin, N. (1998). Comorbidity of Asperger syndrome: A preliminary report. *Autism, 42,* 279–283.

Glass, K. L., Guli, L. A., & Semrud-Clikeman, M. (2000). Social competence intervention program: A pilot program for the development of social competence. *Journal of Psychotherapy in Independent Practice, 1,* 21–33.

Granhom, E., Ben-Zeev, D., & Link, P. C. (2009). Social disinterest attitudes and group cognitive-behavioral social skills training for functional disability in schizophrenia. *Schizophrenia Bulletin, 35*(5), 874–883.

Gray, C. (1994). *Comic strip conversations.* Arlington, TX: Future Horizons.

Gray, C. (1996). "Social assistance." In A. Fullerton, J. Stratton, & C. Gray (Eds.), *Higher functioning adolescents and young adults with autism: A teacher's guide.* Austin, TX: Pro-Ed.

Gray, C. (1998). Social Stories and comic strip conversations with students with Asperger syndrome and high-functioning autism. In E. Schopler, G. B. Mesibov, & L. J. Kunce (Eds.), *Asperger syndrome or high-functioning autism?* New York: Plenum Press.

Gray, C. (2000). *The new Social Story book.* Arlington, TX: Future Horizons.

Greco, L. A., & Morris, T. L. (2001). Treating childhood shyness and related behavior: Empirically evaluated approaches to promote positive social interactions. *Clinical Child and Family Psychology Review, 4*(4), 299–318.

Greene, R. W., Biederman, J., Faraone, S. V., Wilens, T. E:, Mick, E., & Blier, H. K. (1999). Further validation of social impairment as a predictor of substance use disorders: Findings from a sample of siblings of boys with and without ADHD. *Journal of Clinical Child Psychology, 28,* 349–354.

Gresham, F. M., & Elliott, S. N. (1990). *Social skills rating system.* Circle Pines, MN: American Guidance Service.

Gresham, F. M., Sugai, G., & Horner, R. H. (2001). Interpreting outcomes of social skills training for students with high-incidence disabilities. *The Council for Exceptional Children, 67,* 331–344.

Gresham, F. M., Thomas, A., & Grimes, J. (2002). Best practices in social skills training. In *Best practices in school psychology IV* (Vol. 2, pp. 1029–1040). Washington, DC: National Association of School Psychologists.

Gutstein, S. E., & Whitney, T. (2002). Asperger syndrome and the development of social competence. *Focus on Autism and Other Developmental Disabilities, 17*(3), 161–171.

Hanley, G. P., Iwata, B. A., & McCord, B. (2003). Functional analysis of problem behavior: A review. *Journal of Applied Behavior Analysis, 36,* 147–185.

Hansen, D. J., Nangle, D. W., & Meyer, K. A. (1998). Enhancing the effectiveness of social skills interventions. *Education and Treatment of Children, 21,* 489–513.

Happe, F. G. (1996). Studying weak central coherence at low levels: Children with autism do not succumb to visual illusions: A research note. *Journal of Child Psychology and Psychiatry, 37,* 873–877.

Haring, T., Breen, C., Weiner, J., Kennedy, C., & Bednersh, E. (1995). Using videotape modeling to facilitate generalized purchasing skills. *Journal of Behavioral Education, 5,* 29–53.

Harrower, J. K., & Dunlap, G. (2001). Including children with autism in general education classrooms: A review of effective strategies. *Behavior Modification, 25,* 762–784.

Herbert, J. D., Gaudiano, B. A., Rheingold, A. A., Myers, V. H., Dalrymple, K., & Nolan, E. M. (2005). Social skills training augments the effectiveness of cognitive behavioral group therapy for social anxiety disorder. *Behavior Therapy, 36*(2), 125–138.

Howlin, P., Baron-Cohen, S., & Hadwin, J. (1999) *Teaching children with autism to mindread: A practical guide.* Chichester, UK: Wiley.

Howlin, P., Goode, J., Hutton, J., & Rutter, M. (2004). Adult outcome for children with autism. *Journal of Child Psychology and Psychiatry, 45,* 212–229.

Hutton, J., Goode, S., Murphy, M., Le Couteur, A., & Rutter, M. (2008). New-onset psychiatric disorders in individuals with autism. *Autism, 12,* 373–390.

Iwata, B. A., Dorsey, M. F., Slifer, K. J., Bauman, K. E., & Richman, G. S. (1982). Toward a functional analysis of self-injury. *Analysis and Intervention in Developmental Disabilities, 2,* 3–20.

Johnson, C. R., Handen, B. J., Butter, E., Wagner, A., Mulick, J., Sukhodolsky, D. G., et al. (2007). Development of a parent training program for children with pervasive developmental disorders. *Behavioral Interventions, 22,* 201–221.

Kamps, D. M., Barbetta, P. M., Leonard, B. R., & Delquadri, J. (1994). Classwide peer tutoring: An integration strategy to improve reading skills and promote peer interactions among students with autism and general education peers. *Journal of Applied Behavior Analysis, 27,* 49–61.

Kelly, A. B., Garnett, M. S., Attwood, T., & Peterson, C. (2008). Autism spectrum symptomatology in children: The impact of family and peer relationships. *Journal of Abnormal Child Psychology, 36,* 1069–1081.

Kendall, P. C., & Suveg, C. (2006). Treating anxiety disorders in youth. In P. C. Kendall (Ed.), *Child and adolescent therapy: Cognitive-behavioral procedures* (3rd ed., pp. 243–294). New York: Guilford Press.

Klin, A., Jones, W., Schultz, R., & Volkmar, F. (2003). The enactive mind—from actions to cognition: Lessons from autism. In D. J. Cohen & F. R. Volkmar (Eds.), *Handbook of autism and pervasive developmental disorders* (2nd ed., pp. 682–704). New York: Wiley.

Klin, A., Jones, W., Schultz, R., Volkmar, F. R., & Cohen, D. J. (2002). Visual fixation patterns during viewing of naturalistic social situations as predictors of social competence in individuals with autism. *Archives of General Psychiatry, 59*, 809–816.

Koegel, L. K., Koegel, R. L., & Brookman, L. I. (2005). Child-initiated interactions that are pivotal in intervention for children with autism. In E. D. Hibbs (Eds.), *Psychosocial treatments for child and adolescents disorders: Empirically based strategies for clinical practice* (2nd ed., pp. 633–657). Washington, DC: American Psychological Association.

Koegel, L. K., Koegel, R. L., Hurley, C., & Frea, W. D. (1992). Improving social skills and disruptive behavior in children with autism through self-management. *Journal of Applied Behavior Analysis, 25*, 341–353.

Krantz, P. J., & McClannahan, L. E. (1993). Teaching children with autism to initiate with peers: Effects of a script-fading procedure. *Journal of Applied Behavior Analysis, 26*, 121–132.

Kuusikko, S., Pollock-Wurman, R., Jussila, K., Carter, A.S., Mattila, M., Ebieling, H., et al. (2008). Social anxiety in high-functioning children and adolescents with autism and Asperger syndrome. *Journal of Autism and Developmental Disorders, 38*, 1697–1709.

Laushey, K. M., & Heflin, L. J. (2000). Enhancing social skills of kindergarten children with autism through the training of multiple peers as tutors. *Journal of Autism and Developmental Disorders, 30*, 183–193.

LeBlanc, L. A., Coates, A. M., Daneshvar, S., Charlop-Christy, M. H., Morris, C, & Lancaster, B. M. (2003). Using video modeling and reinforcement to teach perspective-taking skills to children with autism. *Journal of Applied Behavior Analysis, 36*, 253–257.

LeGoff, D. B. (2004). Use of LEGO as a therapeutic medium for improving social competence. *Journal of Autism and Developmental Disorders, 34*, 557–571.

Lopata, C., Thomeer, M. L., Volker, M. A., & Nida, R. E. (2006). Effectiveness of a cognitive-behavioral treatment on the social behaviors of children with Asperger disorder. *Focus on Autism and Other Developmental Disabilities, 21*, 237–244.

Marans, W. D., Rubin, E., & Laurent, A. (2000). Addressing social communication skills in individuals with high-functioning autism and Asperger syndrome: Critical priorities in educational programming. In D. J. Cohen & F. R. Volkmar (Eds.), *Handbook of autism and pervasive developmental disorders* (2nd ed., pp. 977–1002). New York: Wiley.

Martin, A., Koenig, K., Anderson, G. M., & Scahill, L. (2003). Low-dose fluvoxamine treatment of children and adolescents with pervasive developmental disorders: A prospective, open-label study. *Journal of Autism and Developmental Disorders, 33*(1), 77–85.

Matson, J. L., & Nebel-Schwalm, M. S. (2007). Comorbid psychopathology with autism spectrum disorder in children: An overview. *Research in Developmental Disabilities, 28*(4), 341–352.

McClannahan, L. E., & Krantz, P. J. (2005). *Teaching conversation to children with autism: Scripts and script fading.* Bethesda, MD: Woodbine House.

McConnell, S. R. (2002). Interventions to facilitate social interaction for young children with autism: Review of available research and recommendations for educational intervention and future research. *Journal of Autism and Developmental Disorders, 32,* 351–372.

McCoy, K., & Hermansen, E. (2007). Video modeling for individuals with autism: A review of model types and effects. *Education and Treatment of Children, 30,* 183–213.

Morton, J. F., & Campbell, J. M. (2008). Information source affects peers' initial attitudes toward autism. *Research in Developmental Disabilities, 29,* 189–201.

Mulick, J. A., & Butter, E. M. (2002). Educational advocacy for children with autism. *Behavioral Interventions, 17,* 57–74.

Mueser, K. T., & Bellack, A. S. (2007). Social skills training: Alive and well? *Journal of Mental Health, 16*(5), 549–552.

Munesue, T., Ono, Y., Mutoh, K., Shimoda, K., Nakatani, H., & Kikuchi, M. (2008). High prevalence of bipolar disorder comorbidity in adolescents and young adults with high-functioning autism spectrum disorder: A preliminary study of 44 outpatients. *Journal of Affective Disorders, 111,* 170–175.

Myles, B. (2003). Behavioral forms of stress management for individuals with Asperger syndrome. *Child and Adolescent Psychiatric Clinics of North America, 12,* 123–141.

Myles, B., Barnhill, G., Hagiwara, T., Griswold, D., & Simpson, R. (2001). A synthesis of studies on the intellectual, academic, social/emotional and sensory characteristics of children with Asperger syndrome. *Education and Training in Mental Retardation and Developmental Disabilities, 36,* 304–311.

Nangle, D. W., Erdley, C. A., Carpenter, E. M., & Newman, J. E. (2002). Social skills training as a treatment for aggressive children and adolescents: A developmental-clinical integration. *Aggression and Violent Behavior, 7*(2), 169–199.

Nikopoulos, C. K., & Keenan, M. (2007). Using video modeling to teach complex social sequences to children with autism. *Journal of Autism and Developmental Disorders, 37,* 678–693.

Owens, G., Granader, Y., Humphrey, A., & Baron-Cohen, S. (2008). LEGO therapy and the social use of language programme: An evaluation of two social skills interventions for children with high functioning autism and Asperger syndrome. *Journal of Autism and Developmental Disorders, 38*(10), 1944–1957.

Ozonoff, S. (1997). Causal mechanisms of autism: Unifying perspectives from an information-processing framework. In D. J. Cohen & F. R. Volkmar

(Eds.), *Handbook of autism and pervasive developmental disorders* (2nd ed., pp. 868–879). New York: Wiley.

Ozonoff, S., Dawson, G., & McPartland, J. (2002). *A parent's guide to Asperger syndrome and high functioning autism: How to meet the challenges and help your child thrive*. New York: Guilford Press.

Ozonoff, S., & Jensen, J. (1999). Brief report: Specific executive function profiles in three neurodevelopmental disorders. *Journal of Autism and Developmental Disorders, 29*, 171–177.

Parker, J. G., & Asher, S. R. (1987). Peer relations and later personal adjustment: Are low-accepted children at risk? *Psychological Bulletin, 102, 357–389.*

Pennington, B. F., & Ozonoff, S. (1996). Executive functions and developmental psychopathology. *Journal of Child Psychology and Psychiatry, 37*, 51–87.

Research Units on Pediatric Psychopharmacology Autism Network (RUPP). (2002). Risperidone in children with autism and serious behavioral problems. *New England Journal of Medicine, 347*, 314–321.

Research Units on Pediatric Psychopharmacology Autism Network (RUPP). (2005). Randomized, controlled, crossover trial of methylphenidate in pervasive developmental disorders with hyperactivity. *Archives of General Psychiatry, 62*, 1266–1274.

Research Units on Pediatric Psychopharmacology Autism Network (RUPP). (2007). Parent training for children with pervasive developmental disorders: A multi-site feasibility trial. *Behavioral Interventions, 22*, 179–199.

Rocha, M. L., Schreibman, L., & Stahmer, A. C. (2007). Effectiveness of training parents to teach joint attention in children with autism. *Journal of Early Intervention, 29*(2), 154–172.

Rogers, S. J. (2000). Interventions that facilitate socialization in children with autism. *Journal of Autism and Developmental Disorders, 30*, 399–409.

Sansosti, F. J. & Powell-Smith, K. A. (2006). Using social stories to improve the social behavior of children with asperger syndrome. *Journal of Positive Behavior Interventions, 8*(1), 43–57.

Sansosti, F. J., & Powell-Smith, K. A. (2008). Using computer-presented Social Stories and video models to increase the social communication skills of children with High-Functioning Autism Spectrum Disorders. *Journal of Positive Behavior Interventions, 10*(3), 162–178.

Schopler, E., & Mesibov, G. (1983). *Autism in adolescents and adults*. New York: Plenum Press.

Schreibman, L. (2000). Intensive behavioral/psychoeducational treatments for autism: Research needs and future directions. *Journal of Autism and Developmental Disorders, 30*, 373–378.

Segrin, C. (2000). Social skills deficits associated with depression. *Clinical Psychology Review, 20*(3), 379–403.

Segrin, C., & Givertz, M. (2003). Methods of social skills training and development. In J.O. Greene & B.R. Burleson (Eds.), *Handbook of communication and social interaction skills* (pp. 135–178). Mahwah, NJ: Erlbaum.

Sigman, M., & Ruskin, E. (1999). Continuity and change in the social competence of children with autism, Down syndrome, and developmental delays.

Monographs of the Society for Research in Child Development, 64(1, Serial No. 256, pp. v–vi). Malden, MA: Blackwell Publishers.

South, M., Ozonoff, S., & McMahon, W. M. (2007). The relationship between executive functioning, central coherence, and repetitive behaviors in the high-functioning autism spectrum. *Autism, 11*, 437–451.

Spence, S. H. (2003). Social skills training with children and young people: Theory, evidence and practice. *Child and Adolescent Mental Health, 8*, 84–96.

Sterling, L., Dawson, G., Estes, A., & Greenson, J. (2008). Characteristics associated with presence of depressive symptoms in adults with autism spectrum disorder. *Journal of Autism and Developmental Disorders, 38*, 1011–1018.

Sturm, H., Fernell, E., & Gillberg, C. (2004). Autism spectrum disorders in children with normal intellectual levels: Associated impairments and subgroups. *Developmental Medicine and Child Neurology, 46*, 444–447.

Sze, K. M., & Wood J. J. (2007). Cognitive behavioral treatment of comorbid anxiety disorders and social difficulties in children with high-functioning autism: A case report. *Journal of Contemporary Psychotherapy, 37*, 133–143.

Tantam, D. (2003). The challenge of adolescents and adults with Asperger syndrome. *Child and Adolescent Psychiatric Clinics of North America, 12*, 143–163.

Tenhula, W. N., & Bellack, A. S. (2008). Social skills training. In K. T. Mueser & D. V. Jeste (Eds.), *Clinical handbook of schizophrenia* (pp. 240–248). New York: Guilford Press.

Thede, L. L., & Coolidge, F. L. (2007). Psychological and neurobehavioral comparisons of children with Asperger's disorder versus high-functioning autism. *Journal of Autism and Developmental Disorders, 37*(5), 847–854.

Twachtman-Cullen, D. (1998). Language and communication in high-functioning autism and Asperger syndrome. In E. Schopler, G. B. Mesibov, & L. J. Kunce (Eds.), *Asperger syndrome or high-functioning autism?* (pp. 199–225). New York: Plenum Press.

Vismara, L. A., Gengoux, G. W., Boettcher, M., Koegel, R. L., & Koegel, L. K. (2006). *Facilitating play dates for children with autism and typically developing peers in natural settings: A training manual.* Santa Barbara: University of California Press.

Wainscot, J. J., Naylor, P., Sutcliffe, P., Tantam, D., & Williams, J. V. (2008). Relationships with peers and use of the school environment of mainstream secondary school pupils with Asperger syndrome (high-functioning autism): A case-control study. *International Journal of Psychology and Psychological Therapy, 8*, 25–38.

White, S. W., Koenig, K., & Scahill, L. (2007). Social skills development in children with autism spectrum disorders: A review of the intervention research. *Journal of Autism and Developmental Disorders, 37*, 1858–1868.

White, S. W., Koenig, K., & Scahill, L. (2010). Group therapy to improve social skills in adolescents with high-functioning autism spectrum disorders. *Focus on Autism and Other Developmental Disabilities, 25*(4), 209–219.

White, S. W., Oswald, D., Ollendick, T., & Scahill, L. (2009). Anxiety in children and adolescents with autism spectrum disorders. *Clinical Psychology Review, 29*(3), 216–229.

Williams, S. K., Johnson, C., & Sukhodolsky, D. G. (2005). The role of the school psychologist in the inclusive education of school-age children with autism spectrum disorders. *Journal of School Psychology, 43*, 117–136.

Index

Pages followed by an *f* or *t* indicate figures or tables.

177